Pediatrician

International Journal of Child and Adolescent Health

Founded 1858 as 'Jahrbuch für Kinderheilkunde und physische Erziehung', continued as 'Annales Paediatrici' (1938–1966), 'Pediatric Research' (1967–1970) and 'Paediatrician' (1972–1982)

General Information

Publication data: 'Pediatrician' is published 4 times annually. Volume 17 with 4 issues appears in 1990.

Subscription rates: Subscriptions run for a full calendar year. Prices are given per volume, surface postage included.

Personal subscription: SFr. 94.–, US$ 57.50. (Must be in the name of, billed to, and paid by an individual. Order must be marked 'personal subscription'.)

Institutional subscription: SFr. 188.–, US$ 115.00. (Regular rate.)

Airmail postage: SFr. 25.–, US$ 18.00. (Extra per volume.)

Microform subscription: SFr. 94.–, US$ 57.50. (Available exclusively to subscribers of the paper edition.)

Single issues and back volumes: Information on availability and prices can be obtained through the Publisher.

Subscription orders: Orders can be placed at agencies, bookstores, directly with the Publisher S. Karger AG, P.O. Box, CH–4009 Basel (Switzerland) or with any of the following distributors:

Deutschland, West-Berlin, Österreich, Ost-Europa: S. Karger GmbH, Postfach 1724 D–8034 Germering/München

France: Librairie Luginbühl 36, bd de Latour-Maubourg, F–75007 Paris

Great Britain, Ireland: S. Karger Publishers, 1 Torberry Drive Petersfield, Hampshire GU 31 4HW

USA: S. Karger Publishers, Inc. 26 West Avon Road, P.O. Box 529 Farmington, CT 06085

India, Bangladesh, Sri Lanka: S. Karger India Subscription Agency B–5/132 Safdarjung Enclave New Delhi-110029

Japan: Katakura Libri, Inc. 36-9 Hongo 3-chome, Bunkyo-ku, Tokyo 113

Change of address: Both old and new address should be stated and sent to the subscription source.

Bibliographic indices: This journal is regularly listed in bibliographic services.

Advertising: Correspondence and rate requests should be addressed to the Publisher.

KARGER

Pediatrician
Printed in Switzerland

S. Karger AG,
Postfach, CH–4009 Basel (Schweiz)

Erscheint vierteljährlich
pro Jahr 1 Band zu 4 Heften

Pediatrician

Submission: Only original papers written in English are considered and should be sent to:

D.W. Kaplan, MD, MPH
The Children's Hospital
1056 East 19th Avenue
Denver, CO 80218 (USA)

Manuscripts should be submitted in triplicate (with three sets of illustrations of which one is an original), typewritten double-spaced on one side of the paper, with a wide margin.

Conditions: All manuscripts are subject to editorial review. Manuscripts are received with the explicit understanding that they are not under simultaneous consideration by any other publication. Submission of an article for publication implies the transfer of the copyright from the author to the publisher upon acceptance. Accepted papers become the permanent property of 'Pediatrician' and may not be reproduced by any means, in whole or in part, without the written consent of the publisher. It is the author's responsibility to obtain permission to reproduce illustrations, tables, etc. from other publications.

Arrangement:

Title page: The first page of each paper should indicate the title (main title underlined), the authors' names, and the institute where the work was conducted. A short title for use as running head is also required.

Key words: For indexing purposes, a list of 3–10 key words in English is essential.

Abstract: Each paper needs an abstract of up to 250 words.

Small type: Paragraphs which can or must be set in smaller type (case histories, test methods, etc.) should be indicated with a 'p' (petit) in the margin on the left-hand side.

Footnotes: Avoid footnotes. When essential, they are numbered consecutively and typed at the foot of the appropriate page.

Tables and illustrations: Tables and illustrations (both numbered in Arabic numerals) should be prepared on separate sheets. Tables require a heading and figures a legend, also prepared on a separate sheet. For the reproduction of illustrations, only good drawings and original photographs can be accepted; negatives or photocopies cannot be used. When possible, group several illustrations on one block for reproduction (max. size 176 × 224 mm) or provide crop marks. On the back of each illustration, indicate its number, the author's name, and 'top'. Color illustrations are reproduced at the author's expense.

References: In the text identify references by Arabic numerals [in square brackets]. Material submitted for publication but not yet accepted should be noted as 'unpublished data' and not be included in the reference list. The list of references should include only those publications which are cited in the text. Do not alphabetize; number references in the order in which they are first mentioned in the text. The surnames of the authors followed by initials should be given. There should be no punctuation other than a comma to separate the authors. Cite all authors, 'et al' is not sufficient. Abbreviate journal names according to the Index Medicus system. (Also see International Committee of Medical Journal Editors: Uniform requirements for manuscripts submitted to biomedical journals. Br Med J 1988;296:401–405.)

Examples

(a) Papers published in periodicals: Kauffman HF, van der Heide S, Beaumont F, Blok H, de Vries K: Class-specific antibody determination against *Aspergillus fumigatus* by means of the enzyme-linked immunosorbent assay. III. Comparative study: IgG, IgA, IgM ELISA titers, precipitating antibodies and IgE binding after fractionation of the antigen. Int Arch Allergy Appl Immunol 1986;80:300–306.

(b) Monographs: Matthews DE, Farewell VT: Using and Understanding Medical Statistics. Basel, Karger, 1985.

(c) Edited books: Hardy WD Jr, Essex M: FeLV-induced feline acquired immune deficiency syndrome: A model for human AIDS; in Klein E (ed): Acquired Immunodeficiency Syndrome. Prog Allergy. Basel, Karger, 1986, vol 37, pp 353–376.

Full address: The exact postal address complete with postal code of the senior author must be given. If correspondence is handled by someone else, indicate this accordingly.

Further details: Authors may consult our leaflet 'Rules for the Preparation of Manuscripts', available on request from the Publisher, S. Karger AG, P.O. Box, CH–4009 Basel (Switzerland).

Galley proofs: Unless indicated otherwise, galley proofs are sent to the first-named author and should be returned with the least possible delay. Alterations made in galley proofs, other than the correction of printer's errors, are charged to the author. No page proofs are supplied.

Reprints: Order forms and a price list are sent with the galley proofs. Orders submitted after the issue is printed are subject to considerably higher prices. Allow five weeks from date of publication for delivery of reprints.

KARGER

Perspectives in Pediatric Pathology (ISSN 0091–2921), **Vol. 13**
Series Editors: H.S. Rosenberg, Houston, Tex.; J. Bernstein, Royal Oak, Mich.

Organ Transplantation in Children

Editors:

C.R. Abramowsky, Cleveland, Ohio;

R.B. Colvin, Boston, Mass.

The five expert review articles in this book offer a state-of-the-art account of present-day practices in pediatric organ transplantation. Opening with a dedication to Le Tan Vinh, one of the founders of pediatric pathology, following chapters focus on general principles, applications and common complications associated with transplantation of bone marrow and other organs such as the liver, heart, lung and kidney in children. Furthermore, the pathologic consequences of immunosuppressive therapy to avoid transplant rejection are discussed in detail.
An excellent and authoritative overview of organ transplantation, this book is a valuable resource for pediatric surgeons, pathologists, and pharmacologists as well as for students of pediatrics and surgery who wish to profit from the original experiences of leading specialists in the field.

Fields of Interest

Pathology; Pediatrics; Surgery; Pharmacology, Transplantation

Contents

Perspectives in Pediatric Pathology, Vol. 13
Organ Transplantation in Children
Editors: Abramowsky, C.R. (Cleveland, Ohio); Colvin, R.B. (Boston, Mass.)
VIII + 206 p., 112 fig., 20 tab., hard cover, 1989
SFr. 228.– / DM 273.– / £ 99.20 / US$ 169.00
US$ price for USA, £ price for UK only (subject to change)
ISBN 3–8055–5019–7

KARGER

KI 89738

Recent Achievements in Restorative Neurology (ISSN 1013–7467), **Vol. 3**
Series Editor: M.R. Dimitrijević, Houston, Tex.

Editors: M.R. Dimitrijević, Houston, Tex.; P.D. Wall, London; U. Lindblom, Stockholm

Altered Sensation and Pain

Chronic neurological pain and altered sensation resulting from disorders of the central or peripheral nervous system are among the unsolved practical problems facing contemporary neurology. These two categories of painful experience were the theme of an international symposium aimed at advancing the practice of restorative neurology. Papers in this volume illustrate how new methods for the assessment and classification of pain and altered sensation contribute to a better understanding of the mechanisms underlying nervous system dysfunction. A comprehensive review of the achievements of experimental neurobiology to date in the exploration of these underlying mechanisms is provided, and the efficacy of new restorative procedures to control and modify altered sensation and pain is discussed.
The stimulating exchange of ideas and experience by leading specialists makes this book valuable reading for neurologists, neurosurgeons, and those involved in the rehabilitation of patients suffering from pain.

Fields of Interest

Neurology, Neurosurgery; Rehabilitation

Contents

Recent Achievements in Restorative Neurology, Vol. 3
Altered Sensation and Pain
Symposium on Altered Sensation and Pain, Houston, Tex., November 1988
Editors: Dimitrijević, M.R. (Houston, Tex.); Wall, P.D. (London); Lindblom, U. (Stockholm)
XIV + 214 p., 44 fig., 23 tab., hard cover, 1990
SFr. 198.– / DM 237.– / £ 82.50 / US$ 132.00
US$ price for USA, £ price for UK only (subject to change)
ISBN 3-8055-5036-7

Pediatric Rehabilitation

20 figures, 15 tables, 1990

KARGER

S. Karger · Medical and Scientific Publishers
Basel · München · Paris · London · New York · New Delhi · Bangkok · Singapore · Tokyo · Sydney

Drug Dosage

The authors and the publisher have exerted every effort to ensure that drug selection and dosage set forth in this text are in accord with current recommendations and practice at the time of publication. However, in view of ongoing research, changes in government regulations, and the constant flow of information relating to drug therapy and drug reactions, the reader is urged to check the package insert for each drug for any change in indications and dosage and for added warnings and precautions. This is particularly important when the recommended agent is a new and/or infrequently employed drug.

Printed in Switzerland by Thür AG Offsetdruck, Pratteln
ISBN 3-8055-5270-X

Pediatrician 1990;17:211–212

Introduction

Disabled children and adolescents need pediatricians who are willing to coordinate fragmented specialty care. Rehabilitation programs are the latest marketing thrust in the health care industry. Modern health care continues to salvage children who previously succumbed to devastating illness and injury, creating a new challenge to society – the disabled pediatric patient.

This issue of *Pediatrician* focuses on the relatively new field of pediatric rehabilitation and on the contributions of the various health care disciplines to the care of the disabled child. Psychosocial aspects of disability are discussed, followed by papers on several disabling diseases and/or injuries, specific therapy programs, and finally a paper examining the transition of the disabled adolescent to adulthood.

Carlson et al. introduce this issue with a description of a coping model based on developmental stages which can help promote effective coping and growth in disabled children and adolescents. Reentry into the educational system and community life presents a major challenge to disabled children and adolescents. Carney and Gerring emphasize the importance of interagency cooperation and list the features of appropriate educational programs for children recovering from severe head injuries.

New treatment modalities for spastic cerebral palsy enable communication and mobility not attainable previously. Kohn discusses the neurosurgical management of spasticity and the orthopedic treatments which constitute the new trends in managing this neuromuscular disorder. Burns in the pediatric population create yet another rehabilitation challenge. Carvajal's discussion focuses on the need for skilled initial management of this second leading cause of nonvehicular accidental death, emphasizing that successful rehabilitation of the pediatric burn patient begins with proper initial care. The functional outcome of spinal cord injury depends on the injury, training and education, and the proper use of adaptive technology and aids. Massagli and Jaffe describe the comprehensive rehabilitation of spinal cord injury.

From Glasgow, Livingston and McCabe report the cognitive impairment that follows severe head injury, and note that psychosocial recovery lags behind physical recovery from severe head injury. These authors also make the point that a coordinating case manager can integrate the fragmented specialty care received by many children.

Rehabilitation of the injured athlete is the focus of the paper contributed by Thompson, Hershman and Nicholas. Athletic injuries require accurate diagnosis, prompt treatment and comprehensive rehabilitation to return the injured athlete to sports. Management of the injured young athlete focuses on the reacquisition of flexibility, strength and endurance.

Rehabilitation of the disabled child and adolescent requires the collaboration of many disciplines. Highlighted in this issue are the contributions of physical therapy (Eigsti et al.), occupational therapy (Royeen and Gorga), speech therapy (Gardner and Workinger), and rehabilitation engineering (Milner et al.). These professions concentrate on increasing function, mobility and communication capacity in the young rehabilitation patient.

Disabled and chronically ill children can benefit from participation in sporting programs and specialty camps.

Page and Pearson discuss the observed psychological benefits of such programs, and provide practical advice on designing specialty recreational programs for disabled individuals.

The disabled adolescent of today must make the transition to the functional adult of tomorrow. Numerous obstacles can make this passage fraught with problems. Thompson describes programs that facilitate this experience.

From birth or onset of disability, the pediatric patient requires rehabilitative assistance to attain the greatest degree of function. Knowledgeable pediatric health care professionals are vital contributors to this rehabilitative process.

David W. Kaplan, MD
Editor-in-Chief
Denver, Colo. (USA)

Pediatrician 1990;17:213–221

0300–1245/90/0174–0213$2.75/0

Psychosocial Aspects of Disability in Children

Carolyn E. Carlson[a,c], *Josephine Ricci*[c], *Yvonne Shade-Zeldow*[b,c]

[a]Cedarville College, Cedarville, Ohio; [b]Department of Psychology; [c]Rehabilitation Institute of Chicago, Ill., USA

Key Words. Psychosocial aspects · Disability · Coping

Abstract. General psychosocial issues must be considered in facilitating the development of children with chronic illnesses and disabilities. A coping model and the developmental stages can be used as a framework to regard the impact of disabling conditions on children and the interventions that encourage psychosocial growth. Health professionals are encouraged to recognize the key role that they can play in promoting effective coping and growth for disabled children and members of their families and to incorporate psychosocial interventions into their practice.

The purposes of this article are to highlight psychosocial processes commonly associated with disability in children and to suggest ways to prevent or lessen psychosocial morbidity. Although much of the information presented may be applicable to children with mental disabilities, the primary focus is on children with physical impairments. Psychosocial variables may influence whether an impairment or disability becomes a handicap.

The authors believe that because the family-child relationship is so important to the child's psychosocial stability, clinical interventions to prevent problems require participation by both children and parents. A model is presented to assess the needs of the individual child and family and to determine interventions that may be appropriate to meet the identified needs.

Incidence of Chronic Illness and Disability in Children

Perrin and MacLean [1] estimate that 2–4% of children in America have severe health conditions that influence daily activities. Gleidman and Roth [2] estimated that more than 2 million children in the United States have a chronic disease or permanent physical disability.

Evidence suggests that children with chronic illnesses and disabilities do have more psychosocial problems than healthy peers. However, the incidence, precise nature and duration of these problems are not well documented [3]. The methodology of many clinical studies is weak, and measures of psychological or social outcomes are absent or cannot be compared because of the lack of common methods of measurement [4].

In an epidemiological study of 3,294 children between the ages of 4 and 16 years, Cadman et al. [3] reported that children with both chronic illness and disability were 3 times more at risk for psychiatric disorders than healthy peers, and at considerable risk for developing social adjustment problems.

Twenty to thirty percent of chronically ill or physically disabled children experience emotional or behavioral problems at some time during childhood and adolescence [5]. This rate is more than 2 times the occurrence in children who are able-bodied and healthy. Despite the increase in risk, Cadman et al. [3] underscore that most children with chronic illnesses and disability do not develop mental health and adjustment problems.

Table 1. Summary of psychosocial issues, coping process and interventions

Stage	Developmental	Coping process			Strategic interventions
		cognitive appraisal	adaptive tasks	coping skills	
Infancy	*trust/mistrust* achieve emotional stability eye-hand coordination sensory discrimination motor skills object permanence eat solid foods	N/A	integrating environmental experience	motor activity (tension reduction and/or goal-oriented) crying, kicking	consistency in nurturing sensory stimulation freedom to move consistent caregiving timely responses to needs verbal soothing clear information to parents
Toddlerhood	*autonomy/shame and doubt* self-control language development fantasy and play elaboration of locomotion sense of autonomy/ asserting independence functional communication interpersonal control	egocentrism (limited ability to imagine alternative viewpoint) questioning through play transductive reasoning	mastery through fantasy and play separation from parent exploring environment increasing communication skills improved frustration tolerance	repetitive activity and play (for mastery and anxiety reduction) protest fantasy comfort time-out experimentation restricting environment	information giving to parents teaching parents care giving and limit-setting skills encourage age appropriate responses acknowledge aggression as healthy response set limits provide safe tension-reduction outlets encourage engaging activities parental/sibling involvement during hospitalization safe havens for parents and children age-appropriate explanation
Early childhood	*initiative/guilt* exploration and mastery independent activity	rudimentary conscience understands right and wrong (views conflict in these terms)	independence develop and identity role in family maintain and protect body integrity	routines ritualized activities	encourage play/fantasy to explore feelings about illness/treatment concise, honest, age-approppropriate information support established routines presence of parents to decrease anxiety
Middle childhood	*industry/inferiority* skill mastery contending with feelings of inferiority peer relationships sensitivity to society expectations	can perceive past/ future consideration of other points of view questions beliefs causal thinking trial and error problem solving	successful productivity peer relationships acceptance	problem solving humor withdrawal aggression control of behavior	use models/diagrams in clarifying information participation in self-direction of procedures enhance opportunities to relate to others with similar difficulties use humor in relationships facilitate maintenance of family, peer relationships during illness encourage responsibilities and chores
Adolescence	*identity* perception of self in eyes of others testing autonomy emotional independence peer relationships body awareness and comfort control positive body image and self realistic future orientation	higher order reasoning propositional logic (formal operations) strategic interventions use of imaginary audience interpretation of earlier experience	reconstruction of experience (reframing, incorporating past) integrating thinking of others contending with self-consciousness competition transition to adult roles successful integration of disability with identity emotional stability independence from parents identify personal identity sexuality separation from peers	repression, denial intellectualization conformity behavioral control motor activity withdrawal	understand perceptions of illness via listening clarify misconceptions encourage and support independence involve in care as much as possible respect need for privacy encourage choice/decision making wherever possible create opportunities for dialogue facilitate peer support opportunities

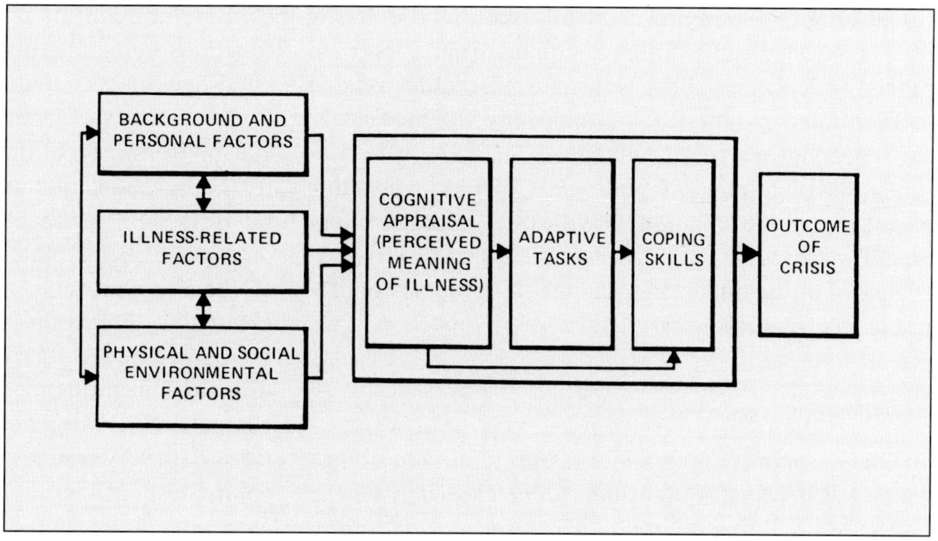

Fig. 1. Model of coping with physical disability [6].

Conceptual Model (table 1)

A model developed by Moos and Tsu [6] to explicate the response to the crisis of chronic illness and disability can be applied to enhance understanding of psychosocial variables related to chronic illness and disability in children. This model is useful in identifying variables as well as for suggesting relationships between variables. It includes three basic elements: the coping process, influencing factors, and outcomes.

Equilibrium is a basic concept underlying the Moos and Tsu model. Equilibrium among physiological systems is essential to survival. When disruptions occur, physiological mechanisms are activated to reestablish homeostasis. Similarly, people need to maintain psychosocial equilibrium. Psychosocial equilibrium is expressed in an individual's behavior which tends to become patterned and predictable. Illness, injury, and the ensuing complications disrupt physiological as well as psychosocial equilibrium. Behavioral disruptions are handled with attempts to problem-solve. When these attempts to restore equilibrium fail, a crisis characterized by disorganization results (fig. 1).

A child with a disability experiences varying degrees of disruption in physiological, psychosocial, and family functioning, depending on a multitude of factors. Disruptions may constitute a crisis for both the child and the family. Often there are repeated crises when new problems emerge, exacerbations of disease are experienced, or the condition has new developmental implications for the child or family. Psychosocial factors are important to consider in the treatment of persons with disability as they play an important role in compliance with treatment regimen and outcomes [1, 7, 8].

Coping Process

Cognitive appraisal is the process of perceiving and attaching meaning to situations and events. For the child or the family of the child with an impairment, this appraisal may include the meaning and threat of the disability, treatment methods, diagnostic tests, attitudes and behaviors of others, and the influence of events on the future. The appraisal process is a key determinant of how a disability will affect a child or family member.

Adaptive tasks are the requirements for adaptation or restoration of equilibrium called for in a particular situation. Moos and Tsu [6] identified two major types of tasks: illness-related and general adaptive tasks. Illness-related tasks include the management of discomfort, symptoms or other incapacitating aspects of the disability. General adaptive tasks include preservation of a reasonable emotional balance, a satisfactory self-image, relationships with family and friends and preparation for an uncertain future. Developmental level will affect the relevance or form that these tasks take. Likewise, there are disease-specific tasks that must be taken into account.

Coping skills include any actions that the individual may use to respond to the adaptive tasks required by the injury. Moos and Tsu [6] identified seven types: (1) denying or minimizing the severity of illness;

(2) seeking and using relevant information; (3) asking for reassurance and emotional support from concerned others; (4) learning about skills and procedures related to the injury or illness; (5) establishing concrete goals; (6) rehearsing alternative outcomes mentally or in conjunction with family or friends, and (7) finding meaning or purpose in the situation. Obviously, age and developmental stage, as well as other variables, influence the relevance of the adaptive tasks and the skills that are appropriate in achieving tasks.

Outcomes

Outcomes of crises or major disruption in physiological or psychosocial equilibrium can be viewed at several levels. Maintaining or improving physical functioning, achieving life satisfaction, accomplishing developmental tasks and developing compliance with a treatment regimen for illness management are a few outcomes that are of concern to most clinicians in pediatric rehabilitation. For the family, important outcomes are family stability, economic stability, and ability to carry out necessary treatments.

The coping process will be negotiated differently by each individual child or family member depending on multiple influencing factors such as those discussed in the following section.

Influencing Factors

Background/person factors include demographic, psychological, physiological, philosophical and religious, and developmental stage variables.

Injury/illness variables include such things as type and location of symptoms, acquired or congenital condition, visibility, prognosis, duration, permanence, and predictability. Each condition is likely to have different psychological meaning and physical and social impact. Shontz [9] identified seven psychological functions of body experience that are helpful in hypothesizing how a given disability might influence an individual child. These normal uses of body experience are as: (1) a sensory register of sensory data; (2) an instrument for action; (3) a source of drives; (4) a stimulus to self allowing for effective use of the body as an adaptive instrument; (5) a stimulus to others which influences expectations and evaluations of others and often determines whether a relationship will develop, a person will be hired, etc.; (6) a private world of experience, and (7) an expressive instrument for demonstrating personal style. Consideration of the impact of disability on these seven functions helps identify specific tasks that the disabled child may have to overcome.

Environmental factors include both physical and social environments of the child, such as barriers to mobility (curbs, doors too narrow for wheelchairs), sociocultural influences, available physical and social resources (economic, social, material), the family and other aspects of the interpersonal environment, and other variables external to the person.

Arrows in the figure 1 model indicate the expected directions of influence of variables. Background/person characteristics influence illness/injury and environmental variables. Variables from each of these influence the coping response variables. Theoretically, variables such as coping style, motivation, emotional stability, goals, and personality influence both the meaning that a situation has to an individual child or family member and the resources available to cope with adaptive tasks. The characteristics of illness or disability, together with developmental stage, determine the adaptive tasks to be accomplished, as well as the coping skills available to a person. Physical and social environments may either hinder coping and contribute to stress or provide resources which facilitate effective coping. A large, available support network provides opportunities for help in accomplishing adaptive tasks, whereas a neglectful or inadequate support network adds stress.

Clinical Enhancement of Desired Outcomes

Understanding the psychosocial issues related to disability enables clinicians to intervene in ways that will enhance coping of the individual child and family members. Perrin and MacLean [1] emphasize chronically ill children have protective factors, as do their healthy peers. These factors include positive parent and child temperaments; cohesive and warm family environments where there are positive parental values and aspirations and reinforcement of the child's attempts to be independent; external supports for the family; supportive teachers, and a peer group. Education about disease, self-care training, social and family support, and promoting success in schools are interventions that have been suggested to facilitate effective coping [1, 10].

In summary, the model is proposed as a useful tool to guide members of the rehabilitation team in their assessment of psychosocial status of individual children and their family members and to facilitate planning interventions. The model represents a cross-section of a situation at one moment in time. Time of injury or illness is an important variable to consider. At what developmental stage was the child when the disability occurred? The discussion that follows enlarges upon the specific tasks of stages of growth and development with emphasis on psychosocial issues, and identifies interventions that may facilitate development of coping skills required to master the adaptive tasks successfully. The reader is directed to literature on specific conditions, as space permits only brief coverage of some general guidelines.

Stages, Tasks, and Interventions

The descriptions below of psychosocial development from infancy through adolescence are based on the works of Erikson [11, 12, 23] on developmental tasks, Kohlberg [13] on cognitive and moral development, Piaget [14, 15] on development of cognitive abilities, Cerreto and Travis [7] on an integrated developmental model for understanding psychological and family factors in the treatment of diabetes, and others as cited. As emphasized by Cerreto and Travis [7], physical, social, and cognitive dimensions of maturation are closely related to each other and the *sequencing* of task accomplishment is more important than the timing of each. Readers are encouraged to read these original works to understand development in greater detail than can be presented here.

Infancy

Impact of Disability/Illness and Interventions

Understanding that infants cry for a reason and that crying should be responded to and investigated in a timely manner is a fundamental strategy for dealing with all infants. Similarly, consistency in nurturing, sensory stimulation, and freedom to move minimize trauma and facilitate the development of trust.

In addition to the physical ramifications are the psychosocial implications for the infant and family. Concerns are many for the family of an infant who is disabled or ill. The parents may grieve the loss of the idealized child and may experience profound guilt [17]. Chronic sorrow may ensue with long-term illness or disability [18]. There may be interruptions in bonding, separation anxiety with repeated hospitalizations, marital discord, financial burden, and stress on siblings. Parents also face the additional dilemma of learning to negotiate the health care system. Health care professionals can help parents to facilitate their infant's maximum potential by offering clear, concise information regarding diagnosis, treatment, resources, and anticipatory guidance.

Toddlerhood

Coping Process

Cognitive Appraisal. The toddler sees the world from his own viewpoint. This egocentricity limits the child's ability to consider that there is another way to view things [19]. The child focuses on one aspect of an object at a time, and thinking is concrete and present-oriented. The toddler thinks in absolutes (i.e. good or bad; hurt versus not hurt). Life and function are related to all objects (i.e. the sun is my friend, so it wakes up every morning and goes to sleep like me every night) [19]. Reasoning is transductive (i.e. illness occurs because he was bad).

The child in this period seems to be in a state of continuous investigation. Play is the life work of the child and occupies the majority of the toddler's day. It is the means by which children explore and learn. Play is also a tool for adaptation. Toddlers play to reduce tension through repetitive motions which lead to mastery of anxiety-provoking situations (i.e. giving 'shots' to a doll during medical play). Toddlers may also use regression, denial, protest behaviors, aggression, withdrawal, fantasy, comfort breaks or time outs, ritualism, and motor activity as a means of coping or to master adaptive tasks [16].

Impact of Disability/Illness and Interventions

The toddler may view his negative behavior (i.e. hitting a sibling) as the cause of his illness or disability thereby provoking fear and a poor sense of self-esteem. Disability may disrupt the normal developmental processes of this stage (i.e. mobility, exploration, separation from parent for short periods of time). Family-child separations may ensue due to repeated hospitalizations.

In a study of mastery motivation in handicapped and nonhandicapped children, Jennings et al. [20] found that both groups were equally curious; however, the handicapped children persisted less on difficult, structured tasks and showed less preference for challenging tasks.

Strategies to help mitigate some of the adverse responses to disability in the toddler stage include acknowledgement of response patterns, encouragement of activities to minimize stress and facilitate adjustment, and provision for safety and privacy. Recognition of defense mechanisms as temporary coping responses enables the clinician to work with family members to help the child move toward age-appropriate responses. Understanding that aggression is a healthy response when under control, clinicians and parents can set limits on undesirable behavior and provide safe outlets (punching bags, therapeutic expression using puppets, drawing of feelings). Gentle touch can convey understanding and acceptance of feelings, and group games and stories may reverse or prevent withdrawal. Parental and sibling involvement in health-related activities encourages family interaction. Stress management activities include rehearsal of potentially stressful situations, time out from actual stressful events, provision of comfort (holding and reassurance) during and after painful procedures, and a safe place where the child can be sure that no painful or frightening procedures will take place. Growth and development can be facilitated by providing safe places for exploration and mobility, age-appropriate explanations, and times of privacy [16].

The impact on the family is much the same as during infancy. Parental coping skills include information seeking, denial, networking support systems, and reliance on faith. Information giving to parents is a key intervention along with teaching necessary caregiving skills. Providing suggestions and support which relate to balancing encouragement and limit setting is important.

Early Childhood

Coping Process

The preoperational child has a rudimentary sense of conscience with basic understanding of right and wrong [13, 21]; the ability to verbalize fears and conceptualize time is limited. Fantasies are prominent and maintenance of body integrity is of primary importance, as are routines and rituals at this time of development. For example, the ritual of sleeping with a night light and special doll or blanket may help to ease the preschooler's fear and fantasy of being eaten by monsters in the dark.

Impact of Illness or Disability/Interventions

Illness may still be viewed as a punishment for bad behavior. There may also be magical thinking such as 'adults could cure if they wished to do so'. Fears of body mutilation are prominent, and treatment may be perceived as hostile or punitive. There is much concern with bodily invasion as with injections, bladder catheterizations or surgery.

Disabilities which limit the child's ability to communicate, explore and navigate the environment (i.e. cerebral palsy, spinal cord injury, ventilator dependency) increase the risk of failure to achieve age-appropriate developmental tasks. Feelings and perceptions of illness, treatment, and limitations can be explored through play, art therapy, and fantasy. Routines and rituals related to eating, sleeping, toileting, managing fears, and other events should be supported when possible to prevent further stress. Focus should be on abilities rather than limitations or disabilities, and the child should be given concise, honest, age-appropriate information about his or her situation. The presence and support of parents and siblings is considered important to allay the child's anxiety.

Middle Childhood

Impact of Illness or Disability/Interventions

The child can use knowledge and understanding of the body, causation of illness, and the process of treatment, and, therefore, needs honest explanations. A sense of self-causation of illness from disobedience or negative behavior may still exist, but may not be easily verbalized. The primary concern is over lack of control of the body and inability to master new experiences. There is still a great need to continue to learn, master, and produce, even during illness. Understanding of death becomes more reality-based: death is recognized as irreversible. Peer relationships and school disruption during hospitalization are of major concern for the child.

Teaching with use of diagrams and models as supplements, and clarification and correction of disability-related misconceptions, is essential. Encouragement to participate in self-care and record keeping and acceptance of the responsibility to direct procedures can ward off feelings of inferiority. Encouragement of exploration among same-age peers with similar disabilities can promote understanding and successful achievement within the constraints of the condition. Facilitating action-oriented activities and peer relationships, being willing to listen and use humor, and providing for safe expression of aggression all enhance a sense of security. Continuation of schoolwork and maintenance of contact with family, peers, teachers and other significant persons during illnesses and hospitalizations will decrease tendencies to withdraw. Family assignment of routine chores and other responsibilities appropriate to developmental stage can decrease the tendency toward overprotection [16] and promote feelings of success and mastery.

Adolescence

Cognitively, the adolescent develops higher-order reasoning ability and is capable of propositional logic. Thus, the adolescent is not bound to considering here-and-now reality but can consider other possibilities [22]. Piaget [14] identifies 'formal operations' as the underlying abilities for propositional logic. Elkind [22] describes reconstruction, the imaginary audience, the personal fable, and strategic interactions as emerging in adolescent thinking and influencing responses to illnesses and disability. Reconstruction of childhood is possible with these higher-level cognitive abilities. The adolescent can imagine what it would be like if aspects of his life were different. Earlier experience may be interpreted differently. In retrospect, a disability in early childhood may be interpreted much more negatively and using a broader context than was possible earlier. Reconstructions, if negative or anxiety-producing, may contribute to new tasks for coping. The 'imaginary audience' is possible because of the new ability to think about another person's thinking. Since the adolescent tends to be focused on personal changes, appearance, and behavior, there is a tendency to think that the imaginary audience is also preoccupied with these things. Such thinking may present itself as self-consciousness. If the individual imagines the thinking of the audience to be negative, depression and withdrawal may result [22].

The 'personal fable' [22, 23] is often a story that we tell ourselves that is not true. The adolescent may reason that since the imaginary audience is watching and thinking about him all of the time, he must be very important. The fable may reflect that 'others may be vulnerable to injury, but not me, I'm special'. Such fables can be positive in keeping persons from constant fear; however, negative effects can occur if needed treatment is refused because of a personal fable.

'Strategic interactions' are competitive. Information is shared or kept hidden to benefit the individual or work to the detriment of others. Such interactions become possible in adolescence. Earlier interaction is called 'frame' interaction, where information is shared in a straightforward way for the benefit of persons involved in the interaction. Elkind [22] asserts that the ability to use both types of interaction makes a third type available: 'strategic manipulation'. This type occurs when one person is using frame rules of mutual benefit, while another is using strategic rules (competitive). 'Two-faced' people use strategic manipulation. Once the adolescent can reconstruct and understand strategic manipulation, he may see relationships with clinicians differently, wondering if they were truly genuine. He is now capable of using strategic manipulation for his own benefit.

Another concept that may come into play during adolescence is 'marginality', defined as difficulty in identifying clearly with a single group [24]. Disabled or chronically ill adolescents may be in double jeopardy with respect to marginality, since they are in transition between childhood and adulthood and may have difficulty identifying with the able-bodied or disabled groups. Wright [25, 26] describes what she calls 'as if' behavior on the part of the person with the disability who tries to act as if it did not exist. The fact of the disability, however, makes it difficult for the individual to identify totally with the nondisabled group.

Coping Process

Cognitive appraisal of one's situation can be much more complex due to the emergence of higher-order reasoning ability, ability to reconstruct situations, use of the imaginary audience, and construction of personal fables described above. The clinician needs to listen and observe carefully to determine how the individual adolescent is appraising his personal situation.

Adaptive tasks include achieving independence from parents, identification of a personal identity (beginning to choose career path; establishing self concept, body image, and sexual identity), and preparing for intimacy in relationships. At this time, individuals tend to solidify their own value system. Depending on the disability and treatment required, the adolescent may have to adapt to separation from peers, change in body image, discomfort, limitations in mobility, and negotiating the health care system.

Coping skills available to most adolescents are many and varied. Defense mechanisms may include regression, denial, repression, projection, displacement, sublimation, reaction formation, rationalization, and intellectualization. The adolescent may use controlling behaviors, motor activity, and cognitive skills to adapt to his circumstances. Conformity with peers is also important in the coping process at this stage [16].

Impact of Disability/Illness and Interventions

Whether an impairment occurred at an earlier stage or occurs during adolescence, the impact on psychosocial functioning can be great because of the many issues involved in adolescence. At a time when the youngster is trying to establish his or her own identity apart from the family, a condition that increases dependency on others can be extremely disruptive. Normal conflicts between independence and dependence may be exaggerated. Body image, self-esteem, and sexuality are of major concern to the adolescent [27]. Those with visible disabilities may feel out of step with their peers. Feelings of denial, anger, depression and fear, which are normal during adolescence, tend to be heightened.

By the time a person reaches adolescence, he or she has many unique characteristics that make generalizations difficult. It is imperative to listen and talk with the adolescent to find out what meaning the disability has for him or her. Adolescents do not easily share their thoughts and feelings with adults. Therefore, clinicians need to be sensitive to subtle and overt cues and encourage interaction with peers. Misconceptions should be clarified. Independence and interdependence, involvement in self-care, and decision making should be supported. Choices should be offered whenever possible. Contact with peers and participation in sports or other reasonable exercise should be facilitated and encouraged. Providing for privacy is very important.

Family Issues

Disruption in family functioning is a potential consequence of disability and associated hospitalizations. Chronic illness in the child often is associated with lowered economic status, increased physical burdens, loss of benefits, and loss of job mobility in families [1]. Families of handicapped children experience high stress levels, are isolated socially and become dependent on helping professionals [28]. Preventing or reducing psychosocial morbidity for parents and siblings often will significantly enhance the child's adaptation to disability-related events. Encouraging as much normalcy as possible facilitates a sense of control for family members. Maintaining a sense of family cohesiveness can be supportive in the context of unexpected or stressful health-related experiences. To this end, strategic interventions oriented toward family members can limit disruptions and enhance family well-being.

Parents need to experience a sense of competence and mastery in the realm of caregiving. Illness or disability, resulting in new temporary or permanent caretaking tasks, may interfere with parental confidence in providing care, as well as pose a threat to the bonding process. At such times, instructing parents in a supportive environment can assist in renewing confidence and competency. Teaching also presents an opportunity for parent-child closeness and a working-through of grief associated with the loss of the idealized child. In essence, a situation rife with the potential for disruption and distance building can be transformed into one of mastery and connectedness.

Waisbren [29] documents the tendency of parents of handicapped children to have increased feelings of uncertainty, helplessness, anger and rejection. Important in contributing to these feelings is the need to be more involved in the health delivery system. Family routines are disrupted considerably, resulting in social isolation at a time when support is critically needed. It is often the tendency of parents under these stresses to establish extreme attachments to the disabled child or to neglect siblings, however benignly. It is helpful to empower the family by 'giving permission' for them to take on other roles separate from those in relation to the disabled child. Such intervention also serves as a positive reminder to the disabled child that no one's needs universally supercede those of others. The communication of disability-related information is helpful to siblings as well as parents. Anxiety surrounding potential changes, new procedures and the like is greatly reduced when facts are available and specific events can be anticipated.

Easton and Gagnon [30] note that a physical disability increases the need for social skills. Indeed, the authors suggest that failure to develop social skills may lead to the creation of 'secondary disability'. Social skills do not unfold naturally when parents and cargivers are focused on the functional aspects of disability. Teaching and provision of opportunities for disabled children to practice are vital to the development of an effective repertoire of behavioral skills. Parents may unintentionally limit the development of these skills due to benevolent overprotection [31], growing social isolation, and lack of emphasis on the importance of these skills by health professionals.

Although a disability can interfere with normal growth and development and disrupt psychological and social functioning, clinicians need to be careful not to build in a negative bias that is transmitted to the child and parents. As noted by Kazak [32], most research on families and children with disabilities has focused on deficits, often omitting ways in which deficits might enhance adaptation or represent strengths in families.

Many families are concerned about the unavailability of respite care, the problems in getting proper medical and educational services, the financial burden, and the emotional drain of a child who is demanding [32]. Policy recommendations are needed to meet these needs at a time when cutbacks in medical, educational, and social programs are the norm. Health care professionals are in a key position to advocate for children with disabilites and to educate parents, teachers, and the community to meet these needs.

References

1 Perrin JM, MacLean WE Jr: Children with chronic illness. Pediatr Clin North Am 1988;35:1325–1337.
2 Gleidman J, Roth W: The Unexpected Minority: Handicapped Children in America. New York, Harcourt, Brace & Jovanovich, 1980.
3 Cadman D, Boyle M, Szatmari P, et al: Chronic illness, disability, and mental and social well-being: Findings of the Ontario child health study. Pediatr 1980;79:805–813.
4 Pless IB: Clinical assessment: Physical and psychological functioning. Pediatr Clin North Am 1984;31:33–45.
5 Lavigne JV, Burns WT: Pediatric Psychology: An Introduction for Pediatricians and Psychologists. New York, Grune & Stratton, 1981.
6 Moos RH, Tsu VD: The crisis of physical illness: An overview; in Moos RH (ed): Coping with Physical Illness. New York, Plenum, 1977.
7 Cerreto MC, Travis LB: Implications of psychological and family factors in the treatment of diabetes. Pediatr Clin North Am 1984;31:689–710.
8 Sargent J, Liebman R: Childhood chronic illness: Issues for psychotherapists. Community Ment Health J 1985;21:294–311.
9 Shontz FC: Psychological Aspects of Physical Illness and Disability. New York, Macmillan, 1975.
10 Turnbull AP, Turnbull HR: Developing independence. J Adolesc Health Care 1985;6:108–119.
11 Erikson EH: Identity and the life cycle. Psychol Issues 1985;1: 18–164.
12 Erikson EH: Childhood and Society, ed 2. New York, Norton, 1963.
13 Kohlberg L: Stage and sequence: The cognitive-developmental approach to socialization; in Goslin DA (ed): Handbook of Socialization Theory and Research. Chicago, Rand McNally, 1969.
14 Piaget J: The Child's Conception of the World. New York, Harcourt, Brace & Jovanovich, 1929.
15 Piaget J: The Origins of Intelligence in Children. New York, International Universities Press, 1952.
16 Vipperman J, McCook-Rager P: Childhood coping: How nurses can help. Pediatr Nurs, March/April 1980, pp 11–18.
17 Solnit A, Stark M: Mourning and the birth of a defective child. Psychoanal Study Child 1962;17:523–536.
18 Olshansky S: Chronic sorrow: A response to having a mentally defective child. Soc Casework 1962;43:191–193.
19 Pontious S: Practical Piaget: Helping children understand. Am J Nurs 1982;82:114–117.
20 Jennings KD, Connors RE, Stegman CE: Does a physical handicap alter the development of mastery motivation during the preschool years? J Am Acad Child Adolesc Psychiatry 1988;27: 312–317.
21 Piaget J: The Moral Development of the Child. New York, Free Press, 1932.
22 Elkind D: Cognitive development and adolescent disabilities. J Adolesc Health Care 1985;6:84–89.
23 Elkind D: Egocentrism in adolescence. Child Dev 1967;38: 1025–1034.
24 Friedman SB: The concept of 'marginality' applied to psychosomatic medicine. Psychosom Med 1988;50:447–453.
25 Wright BA: Physical Disability – A Psychosocial Approach, ed 2. New York, Harper & Row, 1983.
26 Wright BA: Physical Disability – A Psychological Approach. New York, Harper Brothers, 1960.
27 King RB: Sexuality in the adolescent with disability; in McLaurin RL, Oppenheimer MD, Dias L, et al (eds): In Spina bifida: A Multidisciplinary Approach. New York, Praeger, 1986.
28 Kazak A, Wilcox B: The structure and function of social support networks in families with handicapped children. Am J Community Psychol 1984;12:645–661.
29 Waisbren S: Parents' reactions to the birth of a developmentally disabled child. Am J Mental Defic 1980;84:345–351.
30 Easton JKM, Gagnon LR: Psychosocial issues; in Molnar GE (ed): Pediatric Rehabilitation. Baltimore, Williams & Wilkins, 1985, pp 99–120.
31 Boone D, Hartman BH: The benevolent over-reaction: A well intentioned but malignant influence on the handicapped child. Clin Pediatr 1972;11:268–271.
32 Kazak AE: Families with physically handicapped children: Social ecology and family systems. Fam Process 1986;25:265–281.

Received: August 3, 1989

C.E. Carlson, RN, PhD
Associate Director of Nursing for Research and Evaluation
Rehabilitation Institute of Chicago
Chicago, IL 60611 (USA)

Pediatrician 1990;17:222–229

0300–1245/90/0174–0222$2.75/0

Return to School following Severe Closed Head Injury: A Critical Phase in Pediatric Rehabilitation

Joan Carney, Joan Gerring

Pediatric Comprehensive Neurorehabilitation Unit, Kennedy Institute for Handicapped Children, Baltimore, Md., USA

Key Words. Closed head injury, severe · Neurosequelae · Educational reintegration · Public law 94-142 · Interagency cooperation

Abstract. Accidents are the major cause of mortality and morbidity in children over the age of 1 in the United States. Significant numbers sustain closed head injuries severe enough to cause permanent disability and dependence. A critical phase in recovery is the return to school. Many necessary ongoing services are provided by public school systems, but children with neurosequelae of severe closed head injury differ from children traditionally served in special education programs. Smooth transition from hospital to school requires informed participants and interagency cooperation.

Introduction

There are not many events more catastrophic than the sudden and dramatic changes in a child's life caused by severe closed head injury. In the United States, accidents are the major cause of mortality and morbidity in children over the age of 1 with estimates of as many as a half million youth sustaining brain injuries in motor vehicle accidents, falls and sports-related injuries each year [1]. The National Highway Traffic Safety Administration estimates that two-thirds of all infants born today will suffer injuries in traffic accidents [2]. Maryland's 1986 head injury hospitalization rate was 132/100,000 population. Similar to patterns found in other studies, highest incidence was seen in ages 15–24 (237/100,000) with other incidence peaks at age 75 and over (188/100,000) and at ages 0–4 (140/100,000). Severity of injury varied with age. Thus, although 0–4 was a peak incidence of head injury, only 4/100,000 in that age group sustained serious or severe injuries followed by 8/1000,000 5- to 10-year-olds, 12/100,000 10- to 14-year-olds and 25/100,000 15- to 19-year-olds [3]. A severe injury is commonly defined as one resulting in a coma of 6 h or more, or a posttraumatic amnesia (PTA), the period in which the patient is unable to store new memories, of 1 week or longer.

Technologic and clinical advances have led to improved quality of emergency medical services and acute care so that survivors now represent a significant population in need of rehabilitative services. Many of the most severely injured will receive rehabilitative care. However, mildly and moderately injured children and adolescents, and some severely injured, may not receive the benefit of either inpatient or outpatient rehabilitation and in some cases may return home prematurely to the care of their families and the educational system.

Discharge from an acute care or rehabilitation hospital marks a return to normalcy for the severely injured.

Often it becomes a time of confrontation with the realities of physical, cognitive, neuropsychologic, or psychiatric impairments. Recent efforts from the home health care and educational communities to raise awareness and provide professional instruction regarding closed head injury have increased. Still, many children, whose motor function recovers quickly, return to school with no provision of special services because their unseen cognitive, neuropsychologic and psychiatric impairments are not understood. These untreated problems can result in school failure, behavioral manifestations and family turmoil.

The educational community, mandated to serve all youngsters, is faced with a population for whom they are not well prepared and whose pattern of deficits, performance, and progress differs from those they traditionally serve [4].

Outcome

Research in the field of traumatic brain injury clearly supports the causal effects of severe cerebral injury with respect to persistent intellectual impairment and long-term dependency. Chadwick et al. [5] defined their severely injured group as having a PTA of at least 7 days. Persistent intellectual impairment was typically found in children whose PTA exceeded 3 weeks. Those with PTA of 2–3 weeks more often exhibited transient cognitive impairment, although some children showed persistent impairment. Those whose PTA was less than 2 weeks rarely showed intellectual impairment beyond the termination of PTA. Brink et al. [6] studied severe closed head trauma in children who were comatose more than 1 week. Psychological testing performed 1 year or more after injury showed that 33% of the study group were in the normal IQ range, 30% at the borderline retardation level, 23% mildly retarded, 9% in the moderately retarded range and 5% were severely retarded. A direct correlation was found between duration of coma and lower postinjury IQ.

Although approximately one-third of the sample of Eiben et al. [7] of severely brain injured children with protracted coma became independent, almost one-half remained either partially or totally dependent. Patients comatose for less than 21 days achieved a better functional outcome than the majority of patients with a coma longer than 21 days. Parents and guardians identified cognitive and communicative functioning as the major contributors to dependency. Other studies have been more optimistic but have used ambulation and self-care as measures of dependency and have not reported those other, more significant neurosequelae.

Following hospitalization for severe traumatic brain injury, Klonoff et al. [8] found that 25.7% of the study population evidenced school failure or had been placed in remedial classes 5 years after injury. The majority of the children had no previous history of school difficulty. Up to half of the severe injuries studied by Heiskanen and Kaste [9] presented with school difficulties. Those whose coma duration was greater than 2 weeks had the poorest outcome. Academic performance was impaired in the majority of patients of Brink et al. [6], with 76% of those enrolled in school programs assigned to special classes. The more specific focus on reading disabilities of Shaffer et al. [10] found that one-third of children who had sustained compound depressed skull fractures at least 2 years earlier functioned 2 or more years behind their chronological age in reading. Severe reading disabilities were significantly associated with a history of posttraumatic cerebral edema.

Psychiatric disorders represent another prominent area of outcome significant to educational services. Posttraumatic psychiatric sequelae consist of the same behavioral and emotional disorders that affect children or adolescents who have not had head injuries. Pretraumatic psychiatric status, level of intelligence, and psychosocial circumstances should be considered as they increase the risk of behavioral or emotional problems in head-injured children. However, Rutter [11] and Brown et al. [12] found marked increases in psychiatric disorders following severe closed head injury (PTA $>$ 1 week), even without pretraumatic indicators. Approximately half of the patients in the study developed new psychiatric disorders by 1 year following their injuries.

Relevant Sequelae

Neurosequelae of traumatic brain injury fall into three main categories: (1) motor and sensory, (2) cognitive and neuropsychologic, and (3) psychosocial/psychiatric [13]. When reviewing these categories, perhaps the most striking features are the multiple combinations and the variability of deficits. Deficits occurring together may include paresis with disorientation, impulsivity, and decreased judgment, thereby complicating the physical rehabilitative treatment. Sensory impairments, such as a visual field defect, may impact upon the therapeutic treatment needed to regain self-help skills. The frequent presence of combined deficits necessitates that parents, caretakers, and therapists receive enough information about closed head injury to make good decisions about quality rehabilitative treatment.

A rapid and variable pattern of change characterizes the early phases of recovery. Chadwick et al. [5] found recovery most rapid in the first 4 months after severe injury, with substantial recovery continuing for 1 year and progress continuing for as long as 2 years. Although patterns can be identified, it is difficult to describe a typical head-injured child and each child presents a unique educational picture. This variable pattern of cognitive deficits and early rapid change presents a challenge to educational systems. Transitioning back into school requires careful planning and ongoing reassessment of the child and his program.

Motor and sensory deficits include: quadriparesis, hemiparesis, spasticity, ataxia, rigidity, tremors, decreased speed of movement, visual deficits and audiological problems [13]. Prognosis for independent motor functioning is good. As motor deficits are obvious, they are generally identified and physical adaptations can be instituted within the home and community. In the educational setting, motor or sensory sequelae are likely to affect the child's ability to access and fully interact with educational materials and instruction.

It follows logically that cognitive and neuropsychologic deficits affect educational performance. These deficits include: language/communication dysfunction, memory problems, perceptual impairment, tactile sensory dysfunction, poor motor planning, spatial disorientation, difficulties in attention and concentration, poor judgment, impulsivity, decreased ability to abstract, decreased efficiency in learning, and perseveration or rigidity [13]. Although these problems can inhibit new learning, previous learning often remains intact and, initially, measurable academic discrepancies may not exist. Other cognitive sequelae such as poor attention or concentration, impulsivity and decreased judgment are difficult to measure and are not typically considered in school screenings for identification of handicapped students, unless an accompanying academic achievement discrepancy is also documented.

Deficits in the psychosocial/psychiatric domain include: lack of initiative and goal direction, reduced self-image, disinhibition, apathy, social withdrawal, self-centeredness, denial of disability, aggression, immature behavior and family dysfunction 13]. From a child's viewpoint, acceptance among his peers is paramount. Significant problems in any of these areas can lead to peer disapproval and subsequent isolation. Success in an educational setting is dependent upon some degree of self-motivation and self-worth.

Mandated Educational Services

On November 29, 1975, President Gerald R. Ford signed into law the Education for All Handicapped Children Act, also known as Public Law 94-142. This law is a civil rights act protecting handicapped children. Congressional reports at the time revealed that more than one-half of the handicapped children in the United States were not receiving appropriate educational services and many of these children were excluded from public education altogether. Statistics indicate that 4,363,031 children received special education and related services in the 1984/1985 school year [14]. Public Law 94-142 and its companions, Section 504, Public Law 99-457 and Public Law 98-199, currently shape special education practice and procedures. Each state retains an accompanying bylaw encompassing federal standards but including provisions which may vary slightly from state to state.

Six principles are contained in Public Law 94-142. They are: (1) zero reject, the right of every child to a free appropriate public education; (2) nondiscriminatory classification, the right to be fairly evaluated so that proper educational programs can be designed; (3) individualized and appropriate education; (4) least restrictive placement, allowing for interaction with nondisabled peers to the greatest extent deemed appropriate; (5) due process, so that the child or his advocates can challenge any phase of his education, and (6) parent participation in all aspects of their child's education [15]. Eligibility procedures for special education services include a multidisciplinary assessment to determine the need for special education services and to identify a handicapping condition.

Evaluation of a child with a severe traumatic brain injury is usually complicated by the array of neurosequelae that is present. A nontraditional interpretation of findings and experienced clinical judgment is crucial to the identification of difficult to measure deficits that can have a profound effect on educational performance. It is worthwhile for educational systems to refer children, returning to school after severe traumatic brain injury, to private clinicians with specialized experience, as it is unlikely that the school staff has practice with this population.

Handicapped children, by definition, have special education needs arising from cognitive, emotional, or physical attributes or any combination of these. A child's abilities must be impaired to the degree that general education programs have been deemed inadequate. Handicapping conditions include: deaf, hard of hearing, mentally retarded, multihandicapped, orthopedically impaired, other health impaired, seriously emotionally disturbed, learning disabled, speech impaired, and visually handicapped. Characteristics of a brain injured child may not be found clearly within any of these defined handicapping conditions. A physician's documentation that a health impairment has led to the need for an individualized education is often the most reasonable way to obtain necessary educational services. This use of the category 'other health impaired' necessitates a truly individual assessment of needs and educational design.

An individually tailored educational plan (IEP) must be developed for each child. To that end, school systems have developed a range of services through which they hope to provide an appropriate education. A continuum of services should exist in each jurisdiction ranging from individual monitoring of a child's progress (by a special education professional), through various degrees of individual and small group instruction, with residential placement marking the most intensive service offered. Services may vary from state to state but each local educational agency is responsible for providing an appropriate program even if they must look beyond their own jurisdiction for services.

Along with special education instruction related services are required, when necessary, to assist a handicapped child in benefiting from special education. Included are services in audiology, counseling, early identification, occupational therapy, physical therapy, parent training, psychology, recreation, school health, speech pathology, medical services, and transportation. Each related service is mandated only as it pertains to the provision of an appropriate educational program. For instance, medical services are provided only to determine a medically related handicapping condition that results in the need for special education. Medical treatment and ongoing health care are not mandated. Occupational and physical therapy as related services are provided when needed to maximize a student's independence and functional abilities within an educational program. If a child does not need special education instruction, he may not be eligible for related services under Public Law 94-142.

Methodological Restraints to Smooth School Return

Medical versus Educational Systems

After spending time in acute care and rehabilitation facilities, children surviving severe closed head injury are eventually ready to return home. Moving from care in a medical facility to the framework of an educational agency is smooth only if both parties strive to make it so. Too frequently, the failure of the medical treatment facility and public school personnel to identify the differences in their orientations results in delays in services and frustration for families and children who are already physically and emotionally stressed. Optimally, school personnel should be invited to observe the child in the hospital or rehabilitation unit and meet with therapists versed in traumatic brain injury to begin cooperative plans for successful community and educational reintegration. Treating therapists and physicians need to become familiar with the requirements and procedures under which the schools function. Joint regard for the system requirements of all agencies concerned is the first step toward building a working relationship. Sending agencies should identify contact persons in local educational agencies and each may find it beneficial to train their staff in the others' orientation.

School Calendar and Special Services Timeline

Timing is critical in successful rehabilitation yet, by its nature, accidental injury does not afford the luxury of time to plan optimally. School services are infrequent at best during the summer months and vacations. Cooperative efforts and identification of need have prompted a few educational agencies to provide modified summer instruction in special cases.

Along with Public Law 94-142 comes its compliance timeline, meant to safeguard against improper placement of children. Should the schools choose to use the maximum time allotment for each step of the eligibility and placement process, special education implementation could take several months. Knowledge of the process can allow sending agencies to make timely referrals and assist in gathering the necessary documentation, thereby avoiding an interval without appropriate services.

Need for Appropriate Programs

Special education programs are frequently recommended for children who have sustained severe closed head injuries. Theoretically, public educational agencies are mandated to fulfill the needs of all handicapped children. Despite this, there are limitations to the effectiveness of special education for these children. Some survivors of closed head injury do not qualify for services under current state and federal regulations. Although many education professionals advocate special services for these children, their deficits are difficult to measure using traditional tools.

Profiles of traumatically brain-injured students do not fit the accepted notion of learning disabled students as their preserved previous academic achievement is sometimes higher than their measured intellectual ability. For example, a severely injured child may perform age-appropriate academic tasks which have become almost rote but, at the same time, he may display a severe deficit in judgment, reasoning, and the understanding of novel language. The converse, average intelligence with significantly discrepant achievement, is a formula often used to define learning disability.

Even when a child is found eligible for services due to learning disabilities, most special education instruction is designed to remediate specific academic skills. Few provide the intensive cognitive therapy (training in thinking and reasoning skills) necessary after brain injury.

Due to severe behavioral and emotional manifestations, some survivors of severe closed head injury are taught in programs for the seriously emotionally disturbed. The behavioral manifestations of these students frequently have a prominent organic component. A program for the emotionally disturbed may be the best alternative available to ensure the safety and to manage the behavior of these children.

Due to the relatively small numbers of children with severe closed head injuries returning to any one school district yearly, each local educational agency cannot be expected to design a separate program in response to their needs. Instead, local school districts should join in a combined effort to develop regionally based classes designed to address the patterns of deficits and variable recovery rates of these children.

Teacher Training

Due to the relatively small numbers of severe closed head-injured children, this population is only beginning to gain recognition among teaching professionals. Only a handful of texts on exceptional children even mention brain injury and it is safe to say that very few educators have received formal training in this area [4]. Parent advocacy groups have spurred at least an awareness of this population, but ongoing efforts should be made by medical and rehabilitative settings to provide specific training in brain injury and its sequelae to teachers and school administrators.

Noninstructional Barriers

A typical school day is more complicated than just facing those challenges presented during formal instruction. Riding school buses, changing classes, using lockers, selecting cafeteria lunches, toileting needs, physical education and socialization all present their own obstacles to the brain-injured child. These noninstructional demands can prohibit readjustment for a child who may have little insight into his deficits, difficulty in reasoning, memory problems, or is highly distractible. In planning school reentry, sending agencies need to encourage school personnel to examine all aspects of school reintegration including instructional needs, physical management and noninstructional expectations.

Features of Appropriate Educational Programs for Head-Injured Children

Cooperation

As the neurosequelae of brain injury are health-related, educational reintegration is a time when the worlds of medicine and education must mesh. Taking an active and cooperative role, a representative of the medical community can act as an advisor to both the family and school personnel.

Assessment

As assessment is the first step in planning an appropriate educational program, the child and his family should insist upon evaluation by practitioners conversant in brain injury. If the local educational agency cannot provide such expertise, the family should seek private evaluations.

Environment

Brain-injured children may demonstrate persistent deficits in attention, memory, and reasoning. For a child to operate optimally with any of these deficits, a highly structured environment is required. In addition, compensatory strategies addressing these areas should be used. These techniques rely heavily on routine, consistency, and perserverance on the part of both the student and the staff.

Class Size

A small teacher-to-student ratio may be advisable, especially if poor judgment, lack of insight and motor impairment generate safety concerns. In addition, some opportunity for small group or one-to-one instruction should be provided.

Teaching Style

Teachers, by the very nature of their profession, should possess a style of instruction flexible to the needs of their students. Human nature, on the other hand, dictates that people do not always follow their strength of vocation. Although parents cannot be given free reign in selecting a suitable teacher, when possible, school administrators must be encouraged to match the child's needs with a teacher's strengths.

Behavioral Program

Conduct and attentional disorders may require a behavioral modification program. If that is the case, families or advocates should be cautious that these needs are addressed specifically and included in the drafting of the IEP. Behavioral modification can be a tedious and sometimes unrewarding task and is frequently begun in earnest but abandoned before it reaches effectiveness. A nonpunitive, consistent behavioral program with reasonable positive reinforcement intervals (frequent enough to promote desired behaviors) is preferred.

Instructional Emphasis

Whereas most remedial programs address academic skill areas, a corrective program for the brain injured should emphasize process rather than product. Dependent upon the age of onset and extent of injury, many of these children retain factual learning; however, they lack the powers of reasoning and strategies to use this knowledge effectively. Cognitive therapy (or cognitive rehabilitation) is instruction which focuses on fundamental cognitive processes in an effort to enhance a person's ability to coordinate these activities into the behaviors needed to function effectively. For many, this approach needs to be employed both in educational tasks and in activities of daily living.

Providing a student with strategies by which he can become a more efficient thinker is only the beginning of remediation. Generalization to everyday activities is far from guaranteed. Bridging activities which simulate the transfer of newly learned skills to customary functional activities should be incorporated into the educational plan. For example, the integration of learned skills into daily living occurs through outings, field trips, and prevocational tasks.

Integrated Therapies

Related services, such as occupational, physical, and speech-language therapies, have already been discussed. Their availability is compulsory. The manner in which they are delivered is not dictated. For best functional outcome, the related services should be integrated into the classroom or daily living routine as much as possible. This allows the therapist to witness daily demands, the student to practice in context, and the teacher to benefit from added expertise in the classroom.

Teamwork

Parental consent is required at each stage of the eligibility and placement process prior to the initiation of special education services. Active participation of parents in the design of the educational program is preferred. In many cases parents are coming to know a 'new child'. True teamwork between the home and the educational setting can provide the consistency and the continuity needed for successful readjustment.

Reintegration of a handicapped child into the family can cause psychological stress and anxiety for all involved. These children bring to school the positive and negative aspects of their homelife, and these reactions may have a great effect on school functioning. A comprehensive school program should provide support for families when these problems impact upon the child's school success.

Lastly, the school program needs to be assessed as to its willingness to interact with other agencies in the comprehensive care of the head-injured child. Although the system which provides a child's educational management is dictated by demographics, teamwork can and should be fostered. Primary care for the various domains (medical, educational, social) is divided but overlaps unavoidably and thus all involved agencies must work cooperatively.

Case Studies

The following case history illustrates the systemic problems which sometimes arise following severe closed head injury. It describes the events of an unsatisfactory transition to school and community, attributable to lack of awareness regarding the nature of closed head injury and the absence of an appropriate program.

Case 1

Joe was a nine-year-old, accident prone boy with diagnosed attention deficit hyperactivity disorder that had been treated with stimulant medication. He lived with his parents and three siblings. One day, while riding his bicycle, Joe was struck by a pickup truck.

He was flown to a local trauma center where his Glascow Coma Score was 6/15. CT scan revealed bilateral basilar skull fractures and intracranial hemorrhages localized to the right basal ganglion and left thalamus. Joe remained in coma for 6 days. Approximately 3 weeks laters, when he was medically stable, Joe was transferred to an acute rehabilitation facility.

Upon admission to rehabilitation Joe was nonverbal, required maximum assistance for ambulation, and was dysphagic, requiring tube feeding. His attentional problems had exacerbated and he required constant supervision. He was dependent in all activities of daily living because of severe cognitive deficits and asymmetric quadriparesis.

Almost 3 months after his accident, Joe was discharged. He had received intensive rehabilitative therapies and his parents had been trained in his follow-up care. Upon discharge, continued outpatient rehabilitation was recommended. He was still unable to safely eat foods of normal texture and required verbal cuing for safe feeding. His speech was only about 40% intelligible, supplemented by sign language. Cognitively, many skills had returned to the low normal range but academic functioning was in the bottom tenth percentile for age or below for all subjects.

During the latter part of his admission, evaluations and recommendations were forwarded to the school. An initial meeting with school personnel, to ascertain eligibility for special education services, was held the week of discharge. Joe was identified as a multiply handicapped youngster with health-related impairments and learning disabilities. Due to the need for therapeutic feeding, Joe was referred to a multihandicapped center.

Upon review of his records, the administrators of the multihandicapped center determined that their school was not an optimal placement for Joe because he would have no cognitively appropriate peers. An alternate plan to attend a self-contained class for students with learning disabilities for half-days and to receive therapies at the multihandicapped center in the afternoons was devised by the school team.

Three weeks after discharge, Joe began his half-day academic program, but transportation to the center for therapies was not yet in place. After several weeks without treatment, therapeutic feeding was provided through a home-based program at the insistence of the parents.

Following multiple parent contacts with educational administrators and state legislators, Joe finally resumed a full-day academic program, more than 4 months after his discharge. Speech therapy was provided daily, but occupational therapy services were minimal. Joe's special education services were disjointed and did not occur in an organized way. This unsettled situation was a source of great distress to his family and his teacher.

Although academic support was provided in a timely fashion, Joe's teacher was frustrated and sometimes bewildered by Joe's impulsivity and mood swings. There was inadequate parent-teacher interaction and Joe's teacher did not have the benefit of input from other informed professionals. As a result she rejected interaction with the parents and the medical care setting.

Like many families of the severely head injured, Joe's parents have had to become fierce advocates for their son. They now lead the effort for ongoing awareness and training regarding head injury in their community.

For a more successful integration, all levels of educational personnel needed information regarding the nature of this boy's severe closed head injury and the recovery process. This could have been offered by the rehabilitation hospital. Additionally, school administrators should have selected well-suited teachers and therapists, rather than trying to place Joe within one of their existing programs. Lastly, the timing and coordination of services was fragmented and disorganized. A case manager from the school team was needed to direct and oversee the many aspects of Joe's educational program.

Case 2

The return to school was well planned and personnel were well-informed in the following case history.

Sam was 7 years old when he was struck by an automobile while riding his bicycle with his 9-year-old brother. He was transported to a regional trauma center where severe closed head injury and multiple lacerations were diagnosed. On admission to the emergency room, Sam's Glascow Coma Score was 6/15. His cranial CT scan revealed contusions in the left frontal, right temporal and right basal ganglion areas. His coma lasted for 20 days.

Seventeen days after his injury, Sam was transferred to an acute rehabilitation setting. At the time he was still comatose, nonverbal, with inconsistent eye opening, totally dependent for all activities of daily living, incontinent and fed by nasal gastric tube.

Three months later, at his discharge from rehabilitation, Sam was ambulating without assistance and verbalizing spontaneously, but he demonstrated many cognitive and neuropsychologic sequalae of his injury. Sam was operating at the bottom first percentile in cognitive, academic, and language areas. He performed with intellectual and behavioral impulsivity (including aggression), had poor reasoning and no insight into his deficits. Due to these features, Sam required constant supervision and the institution of a behavioral modification program.

Near the end of his rehabilitative stay, evaluations and recommendations were forwarded to his local educational agency for review. One week after Sam returned home, an initial meeting to establish eligibility for special services was held with regional special education coordinators. Sam was identified as a multiply handicapped youngster with both health-related impairments and learning disabilities. A specialized class for brain-injured youngsters, based in a private special education school, was recommended. Time was needed to obtain clearance for state funding to attend a nonpublic school. Three weeks later an IEP was developed and Sam began his school placement with appropriate educational goals and related services, including a continuation of his established behavioral modification plan.

Sam exhibited significant neurosequelae of severe closed head injury and was provided coordinated care from both medical and educational facilities. He returned to a local educational agency acquainted with head injury and an administrative team was assigned to his case. A case manager was identified and a regionally based class was designated as his placement.

Conclusion

The incidence of survival from severe traumatic brain injury is increasing [1–3]. Survivors injured in childhood are often left with both visible motor and unseen neuropsychologic deficits which lead to increased dependency [5–7, 11]. After discharge from acute medical or rehabilitative programs, closed head-injured children return to the care of their families and the local educational agency. Although educational systems are mandated to provide an appropriate education for all [15], the nature of the neurosequelae of traumatic brain injury can make reentry a complicated task. Methodological restraints to smooth school reintegration exist both for the medical and educational communities. Insufficient training and experience with closed head injury, lack of appropriate programs, and the provisions and restraints developed under Public Law 94-142 all affect the ongoing rehabilitation of children with severe closed head injuries when they return to school.

References

1 Frankowski R, Annegers J, Whitman S: Epidemiological and descriptive studies. Part I; in Becker D, Povlishock J (eds): Central Nervous System Trauma: Status Report. National Institutes of Health, National Institute of Neurological and Communicative Disorders and Stroke, Bethesda, 1985, pp 33–45.
2 Christoffel K, Tanz R: Motor vehicle injury in childhood. Pediatr Rev 1983;4:247–254.
3 MacKenzie E, Edelstein S, Flynn J: Incidence and severity of hospitalized head injury in Maryland. Maryland Med J, in press.
4 Savage R: Educational issues for the head-injured adolescent and young adult. J Head Trauma Rehabil 1987;2 1:1–10.
5 Chadwick O, Rutter M, Brown G, et al: A prospective study of children with head injuries. II. Cognitive sequelae. Psychol Med 1981;11:49–61.
6 Brink J, Garrett A, Hale W, et al: Recovery of motor and intellectual function in children sustaining severe head injuries. Dev Med Child Neurol 1970;12:565–571.
7 Eiben C, Anderson T, Lockman L, et al: Functional outcome of closed head injury in children and young adults. Arch Phys Med Rehabil 1984;65:168–170.
8 Klonoff H, Low M, Clark C: Head injuries in children: A prospective five year follow-up. J Neurol Neurosurg Psychiatry 1977;40:1211–1219.
9 Heiskanen O, Kaste M: Late prognosis of severe brain injury in children. Dev Med Child Neurol 1974;16:11–14.
10 Shaffer D, Bijur P, Oliver F, et al: Head injury and later reading disability. J Am Acad Child Adolesc Psychiatry 1980;19:592–610.
11 Rutter M: Psychological sequelae of brain damage in children. Am J Psychiatry 1981;138:1533–1544.
12 Brown G, Chadwick O, Shaffer D, et al: A prospective study of children with head injuries. III. Psychiatric sequelae. Psychol Med 1981;11:63–78.
13 Savage R, Pollack I: An educators manual: What educators need to know about students with traumatic brain injury. National Head Injury Foundation. Framingham, 1985.
14 Tenth annual report to congress on the implementation of PL 94-142: The education for all handicapped children act. United States Department of Education, US Government Printing Office, Washington, 1988.
15 Turnbull H: Free appropriate public education: The law and children with disabilities. Love Publishing Company, Denver, 1986.

Received: August 1, 1989

Joan Carney
Division of Special Education
Kennedy Institute for Handicapped Children
Pediatric Comprehensive Neurorehabilitation Unit
707 North Broadway
Baltimore, MD 21205 (USA)

Pediatrician 1990;17:230–236

Issues in the Management of Children with Spastic Cerebral Palsy

Jean G. Kohn

Maternal and Child Health Program, School of Public Health, University of California, Berkeley, Calif., USA

Key Words. Spastic cerebral palsy · Management · Assistive technology · Multidisciplinary approach · Family focus

Abstract. Management of the child with spastic cerebral palsy is multidisciplinary and family-oriented, with emphasis on maintaining and increasing function and preventing deformities. Assessment, family education, and use of multiple forms of therapy in conjunction with assistive technology will result in optimum outcome. The pediatrician must know about and refer children to specialists who are knowledgeable about management of cerebral palsy. Education, vocational training and preparation for independent or assisted living situations are integral parts of management, and the pediatrician must be aware of community resources.

Introduction

'Cerebral palsy' (CP) refers to a nonprogressive (static) central nervous system motor deficit which may have associated sensory, behavioral and cognitive manifestations [1]. Depending upon the extent of pathologic alterations in the brain, the manifestations may be mild, moderate or severe.

Do we know the etiologies of CP? In spite of extensive investigation, we probably do not [2]. The multivariate analysis of Nelson and Ellenberg [2] in a large prospective study (the National Collaborative Perinatal Project) showed that 'current ability to recognize the important antecedents of cerebral palsy and to predict the occurrence of the disorder failed to account for a majority of cases, and there was an exceedingly high rate of false positive identification. We probably do not know what causes most cases of cerebral palsy' (p. 85). Stanley's conclusions [3] were that 'most of us now believe that the majority of CP syndromes are more like the congenital malformations and intellectual handicap syndromes rather than brain-damage from birth asphyxia or the other perinatal problems. Most authors ... agree that the majority of causes of CP are as yet unknown, but genetic, teratogenic and early pregnancy influences should be pursued' (p. 265).

Has the incidence changed? The incidence has not been substantially altered even with newer management of pregnancy, delivery and the newborn infant [3]. The incidence remains at 1–2/1,000 live births, and 70–80% are spastic in type, with the dyskinesias, ataxia and mixed types constituting the remainder [4]. Management of the spastic CPs is the subject of this review.

If the incidence is remaining essentially unchanged, what about survival? Even in the 1940s and 1950s, it was estimated that 88% of children who survived the neonatal period would live to be adults [5]. Improved survival with better medical care in the past several decades is a reasonable expectation. Thus, the management of children with spastic CP remains an important topic for review.

Terminology and Diagnosis

Spastic CP is classified most commonly by limb involvement: hemiplegia (upper and lower limb on same side), diplegia (major involvement in lower limbs and minor involvement in upper limbs) and quadriplegia (also called tetraplegia and involving all four limbs) [6]. Other forms involving one limb only (monoplegia), both lower limbs exclusively (paraplegia), or three limbs (triplegia) are rare and will be included in the general discussion of management. Associated problems may include speech/language defects, hearing loss, visual defects (especially strabismus), sensory deficits (such as astereognosis in spastic hemiplegia), convulsive disorders and mental retardation. Drooling and swallowing problems, perceptual and visual-motor disorders, visual field defects, and behavior deficits, including attention disorders, may all be a part of spastic CP [7].

Diagnosis is based upon a detailed history, physical examination and laboratory tests. The history follows the usual neurologic patterns of investigation, obtaining information about the family, pregnancy, labor and neonatal course of the child [8]. Physical examination in the very young child is focused on abnormalities of tone, reflexes and posture, delayed motor development and abnormal motor behavior [9].

In spastic CP, hyperreflexia, clonus, increased stretch reflex activity and hypertonus are considered diagnostic signs [8]. Persistent primitive reflexes and failure to develop normal reflexes such as positive supporting and parachute responses are also clues to the presence of spastic CP in infants.

Infants considered to be 'at risk' for CP, due to abnormal history or problems in the perinatal period, should be followed carefully. Since it is not possible to predict with any certainty which children will 'recover' and which will continue to have motor or other problems, it seems sensible to provide services for all children considered to be at risk or to have early signs of abnormal motor behavior. Indeed, in the United States, with passage of Public Law 99-457 (1986), all children with abnormal developmental signs are eligible for educational intervention, which may also include therapies (when written into the Individualized Program Plan) [10]. However, with rapid development of the central nervous system during the first few years of life, many children with abnormal neurologic signs 'outgrow' their CP diagnosis, and caution must be exercised in assessing the 'results' of therapies or other treatments [11].

Laboratory studies may include ultrasound examination in the newborn [12] and brain scanning (computer-assisted tomography) [13], electroencephalograms and electromyograms. Maternal infection as a cause of central nervous system pathology may warrant investigation with screening tests for congenital rubella, toxoplasmosis, cytomegalovirus, and herpes [1].

These studies may indicate the underlying basis of the motor problems, clarify seizure types or provide information about specific muscle spasticity (which may be needed for possible surgical intervention) [7].

Management Issues – Introduction

Families are the major factors in the successful growth and development of children, whether normal or disabled. MacKeith [14] has written: 'The central part that parents play: the support and guidance given to the parents from the earliest time of discovery seems of immense importance (including) the recognition of the importance of stimulation and the encouragement of language development, and that the physical therapy given by the parents, repeatedly, every day, at home is far more efficient than when given by a therapist for half an hour once a week. The eventual outcome for the handicapped person depends on his personality and this derives from the interaction of the child with his parents'.

In the United States, two recent conferences called by the Surgeon General (1986 and 1988) have emphasized parent-centered, community-based, comprehensive care for children with special health care needs [15, 15a]. Components of this care include health care, education, vocational training, mental health services, family support services, recreation and art services [15]. These components need to be organized in a network of services that truly are integrated and coordinated, but the focus of the service system must remain on the family. Families must be included in decision making and in recognizing their rights and responsibilities. The service system must pay attention to the quality of services, appropriate monitoring, assurance of universal access, respect for the dignity of the child and appropriate use of all professionals involved in health care delivery.

Role of the Pediatrician

The pediatrician cannot manage a child with spastic CP alone. The doctor is a partner in the care team, working with the family, therapists, educators and other professionals. The child's normal developmental needs must be kept in mind and the therapeutic efforts must enhance and support development while reducing the adverse effects of the disabling condition.

Physical growth and neurologic maturation interact with functional limitations in the child's performance at any given point in time. However, disabled children's feelings about themselves depend in large part upon the behavior of others, most importantly the family members. Acceptance of the child as a person with needs and desires like those of others, and recognition of the child's capabilities as well as disabilities are crucial aspects of the management of CP. The physician's own attitudes and behavior will convey to the family his or her belief in the value of their child. This is the beginning of effective management.

Components of Management

General Pediatric Supervision

As for any child, usual medical services are required, including immunizations, growth measurements, care of periodic illnesses and sociobehavioral counseling. Unless severe behavioral problems are noted, the pediatrician who knows the family is probably the best individual to discuss developmental and family concerns, as well as to provide anticipatory guidance.

Psychoeducational Assessment and Management

Depending upon the child's performance and sensorimotor developmental activities, special help may be required from psychologists and therapists. Children with visual or hearing deficits frequently will require special assistance. Psychologists, social workers, and mobility instructors for the visually impaired are often a part of the educational system rather than the medical care system. The pediatrician will need to know how to help the family make contact with such professionals.

Orthopedic Management

Orthopedic surgery may be required to prevent and correct deformities, and to improve sitting and ambulation. Orthopedic consultation about orthoses and other assistive supports (walkers, wheelchairs, etc.) also may be needed [16]. Regarding the surgical management of CP, Root [16] has written: 'There is no magic about performing an operation. It requires technical skills, and some experience in decision-making. The art is being able not only to do the operation, but also to put it in the perspective of the total child – the timing of the surgery, to do all procedures at once, if possible, to minimize hospitalization, to limit post-operative cast immobilization and to begin mobilization as quickly as possible after surgery' (pp. 569–570) [for detailed discussion of orthopedic management, see 17].

Neurosurgical Management of Spasticity

Selective dorsal rhizotomy is currently under trial and review in at least 18 centers in the United States. The procedure is performed to reduce spasticity in CP, following reports of successful procedures by Peacock et al. [18] and Peacock and Arens [19] in South Africa. The rationale is that by severing the afferent rootlets, stimulation is reduced to the motor efferents and spasticity is reduced or moderated. Careful clinical research in a number of centers in the United States with preoperative assessment and postoperative follow-up (with intensive physical therapy), is producing early data about the efficacy of this procedure. The criteria for selection of patients and the extent of surgery needed are under investigation. At the present time, however, neither patient numbers nor postsurgical follow-up data are sufficient to offer definite conclusions.

Therapy

Physical and occupational therapies have a long history in treatment of the child with spastic CP. A recent review [20] summarizes the currently recommended therapies and points out once again that there are still no objective measures of success of therapy. Aims of treatment are better patterns of movement, greater postural stability and increased joint range as well as specific activities such as initiation or improvement in crawling, walking with support or bilateral hand use [20]. Neurodevelopmental treatment has been widely adopted, especially for young children, because it follows normal developmental patterns and aims at preparing the child for the next developmental stage [Bobath, 20]. Since this involves knowing a great deal about normal motor development, it is helpful to educate parents for follow-through activities at home.

A major change in therapists' activities in the United States over the past 10 years is their role in assessment and monitoring of activity programs carried out by classroom teachers, aides and adaptive physical education teachers, as well as parents. Isolated therapy programs have evolved into integrated classroom activities, with periodic individual reassessment and revision of programs as needed. Goal-oriented approaches in therapy emphasize assessment of functional activities that the child desires to accomplish and then structuring physical exercise programs toward those ends. This may involve a mixture of therapeutic exercises, assistive devices and adapted physical education with peer groups.

Sports activities may become the mainstay of needed physical exercise in the older child and young adult [21, 22]. In addition to providing maintenance or improvement of physical strength and endurance, sports are a great source of enjoyment and social interaction for disabled youth [23].

Rehabilitation Technology

Rehabilitation technology has been an exciting new addition to the management of disabled children, but it also has introduced new questions: when to introduce technology, how much a child should be allowed or encouraged to use his or her own motor capabilities in contrast to using technology assistance and, if needed, which device to recommend?

Rehabilitation technology includes orthotics (braces), prostheses (artificial limbs), robotics, mobility and seating, and interfaces and controls for devices, including microprocessors (computers) [7]. Assistive devices can provide efficient, functional support, and conserve energy and reinforce the residual capabilities of the child with CP. For the nonverbal child, augmentative communication aids help build language concepts as well as allowing interaction with family and peers.

The array of assistive devices currently commercially available is so large that the problem has become how to match the device to the child's needs. Matching the child's developmental level, functional level and environmental needs is crucial in the selection of appropriate technology.

Orthoses are prescribed to prevent progression of deformity and for support. Newer prostheses for spastic 'tiptoeing' have incorporated features of tone-reducing casts (also called inhibitive casts). Although the research is not conclusive, it appears that posture and ambulation are improved [24]. Orthoses are described more completely in *Orthotics Etcetera* [25].

Seating and mobility devices are prescribed for function and support, but the developmental level of the child is clearly important. Since children normally begin to sit alone at 6–8 months, failure to do so because of spasticity should prompt consideration of seating support, such as a corner chair. Upright posture in a supported position so that hands are free for manipulation of toys is important developmentally. At the normal developmental ages for crawling and walking, appropriate assistive technology should be considered for the spastic child. Early reservations that assistive devices would prevent children from developing their own skills have largely disappeared; children will allow gradual phasing out of assistive equipment as they no longer need it, and some will positively discard such devices as they gain confidence.

Seating support in wheelchairs for older children with spastic CP not only helps to prevent deformity and maintain upright position, but also allows for improved hand function to operate, for example, a power chair or augmentative communication aid. [For further information about seating and mobility devices and where to obtain them, see 26–28].

Assistive and Augmentative Communication Devices

With the rapid advance of the computer age, it has been inevitable that applications for disabled children would be developed. The enormous variety and complexity of these devices have challenged speech therapists as well as rehabilitation engineers to match technology to individual needs. Even very young children (infants and toddlers) can use computers to make choices, demonstrate cause-effect relationships and to control their environment [10]. Vocas, or vocal output communication aids, have been developed for young children as well as older children and adults.

Many classrooms have computers for regular education pupils, and with control adaptations, these computers can be made accessible to disabled children. Again, the concern that use of communication-assistive devices may prevent or delay development of spoken language seems unfounded, and, to the contrary, seems to enhance language and verbal efforts [10]. Most children, in fact, develop a multisystem usage, combining or interchanging facial expression, gestures, pointing with eyes or hands and using the computer systems. [For further information, see 29–34; for listing of computer and control aids, see 35.]

Psychosocial Aspects of Assistive Devices for Children

Assistive technology must be safe, reliable, durable, comfortable, and it must be acceptable to the child and family members. How it looks, and how the child appears with the aid has a good deal to do with acceptance. Most of all, the child must feel that function is improved or that new activities are possible. The ultimate aim is to increase the child's independence and control over his or her own actions. There are amusing anecdotes of children with new powered mobility devices exercising their improved control by 'running away from home' to a nearby playground, or programming 'bad words' into their voice output computers. Normally 'naughty' behavior in disabled children can relieve the need for tantrums or passivity. Being able to control something, whether a toy or a powered mobility device, gives a disabled child a sense of power and competence which may be sadly lacking in other areas. Self-image in a child with disabilities can be improved substantially with assistive technology which is properly suited to the child's needs and developmental level.

Education and Vocational Training

In the United States, Public Law 94-142 (1975) requires every child, no matter how disabled, to receive a free, appropriate public education during years 3 through 21. Public Law 94-457 (1986) extends this education to include 0 through 2 years. Related services which facilitate education also are mandated and may include therapy, transportation, assistance by classroom aides, and the delivery of health care services during the class day. Each handicapped child must have an individualized education plan (IEP) which is agreed upon by the teacher, related professionals and parents, and, when appropriate, the child [36].

Implementation of the two laws has increased integration of CP children into regular schools and classrooms. Bigge [37] recommends that: 'for all children with physical disabilities, we encourage individualized planning with the goal of implementing the overall program that best suits the unique needs and maximum abilities of each'.

Vocational training is a part of the education program for older students, and increasingly has been linked to community participation and work experiences. In a study of vocational status of 60 young adults with CP, the 43 unemployed youth gave as reasons for unemployment the lack of job training and of appropriate work settings. In addition, those youth who *exceeded* their vocational predictions in this study were identified as having strong family support and personal determination [38]. Programs which have been successful in vocational training are described by Wehman [39] and Sailor [40]. The characteristics of family support and personal determination should not be overlooked, however. Curtis [41] concluded from his attempt to place a group of adults with cerebral palsy in employment that the single most important factor was the attitude of parents in the very early years of life.

Independent living programs have been developed in recent years in the United States and may be an appropriate goal even for those individuals who do not obtain employment. Recreational activities, volunteer work and part-time employment also are options for adults with CP and should be encouraged as parents help their teenagers look ahead to the future [for parent reference, 42–48].

Conclusions

Management of the child with spastic CP continues to be multidisciplinary and functionally oriented, with the family unit as the core of consideration. Education and support of the family will pay dividends in the child's long-term performance and self-concept. Pediatricians, orthopedists, neurosurgeons and other medical/therapy specialists can assist the development process by providing appropriate health care. Education and vocational training can provide the skills for competition in the adult world. Rehabilitation technology is an encouraging addition to previously available resources. The final outcome for disabled children is the result of combined professional efforts, family support and their own drive toward independence. As professionals, we must be careful to support that drive, and encourage children's capabilities. We must remember to recognize that the 'person' is much more important than the 'diagnosis'.

Acknowledgements

My thanks to Eugene E. Bleck, MD, for reviewing the manuscript and for his helpful suggestions, and my appreciation to Alice Murata for manuscript preparation.

References

1 Scherzer, A.; Tscharnuter, I.: Early diagnosis and therapy in cerebral palsy (Dekker, New York 1982).
2 Nelson, K.; Ellenberg, J.: Antecedents of cerebral palsy. New Engl. J. Med. *315/2:* 81–86 (1986).
3 Stanley, F.: The changing face of cerebral palsy? Devl Med. Child Neur. *29:* 263–265 (1987).
4 Stanley, F.; Alberman, E.: The epidemiology of the cerebral palsies. Spastics Int. Med. Pub. (Blackwell Scientific Publications, Oxford 1984).
5 Cohen, P.; Mustacchi, P.: Survival in cerebral palsy. JAMA *195:* 462 (1966).
6 Minear, W.L.: A classification of cerebral palsy. Pediatrics *18:* 841 (1956).
7 Bleck, E.; Nagel, D.: Physically handicapped children; 2nd ed. (Grune & Stratton, New York 1982).
8 Baird, H.; Gordon, E.: Neurological evaluation of infants and children. Spastics Int. Med. Pub. (Lippincott, Philadelphia 1983).
9 Molnar, G.: Pediatric rehabilitation (Williams & Williams, Baltimore 1985).
10 Behrman, M.; Jones, J.; Wilds, M.: Technology intervention with very young children with disabilities. Inf. Young Child. *1/4:* 66–77 (1989).
11 Nelson, K.; Ellenberg, J.: Children who outgrew cerebral palsy. Pediatrics *69:* 529–536 (1982).
12 Levene, M.; Williams, J.; Fawer, C.-L.: Ultrasound of the infant brain. Spastics Int. Med. Pub. (Blackwell Scientific Publications, Oxford 1985).
13 Faeber, E.: Cranial computed tomography in infants and children. Spastics Int. Med. Pub. (Blackwell Scientific Publications, Oxford 1986).
14 MacKeith, R.: The restoration of the parents as the keystone of the therapeutic arch. Devl Med. Child Neur. *18:* 285–286 (1976).
15 Gittler, J.: Community-based service systems for children with special health care needs and their families. Nat. MCH Health Resour Cent. (University of Iowa, Iowa City 1988).
15a McCarthy, G.: The physically handicapped child, an interdisciplinary approach to management (Faber & Faber, London 1984).
16 Root, L.: An orthopaedist's approach to cerebral palsy. Devl Med. Child Neur. *30:* 569–570 (1988).
17 Bleck, E.: Orthopaedic management of cerebral palsy. Spastics Int. Med. Pub. (Blackwell Scientific Publications, Oxford 1987).
18 Peacock, W.; Arens, L.; Berman, B.: Cerebral palsy spasticity, selective posterior rhizotomy. Pediat. Neurosci. *13:* 61–66 (1987).
19 Peacock, W.; Arens, L.: Selective posterior rhizotomy for the relief of spasticity in cerebral palsy. S. Afr. med. J. *62:* 119–124 (1982).
20 Scrutton, D.: Management of the motor disorders of children with cerebral palsy. Spastics Int. Med. Pub. (Blackwell Scientific Publications, Oxford 1984).
21 Molnar, G.: Rehabilitative benefits of sports for the handicapped. Conn. Med. *45:* 574–577 (1981).
22 American Academy of Orthopedic Surgery: Sports and recreational programs for the child and young adult with physical disability (Chicago, 1983).
23 Molnar, G.: A developmental perspective for the rehabilitation of children with physical disability. Pediat. Ann. *17:* 766–776 (1988).
24 Taylor, C.; Harris, S.: Effects of ankle-foot orthoses on functional motor performance in a child with spastic diplegia. Am. J. occup. Ther. *40:* 492–494 (1986).
25 Redford, J.: Orthotics etcetera; 3rd ed. (Williams & Wilkins, Baltimore 1986).
26 Bergen, A.; Colangello, C.: Positioning the client with CNS deficits: the wheelchair and other adapted equipment (Valhalla Rehabilitation Publications, New York 1982).
27 Ward, D.: Positioning the handicapped child for function; 2nd ed. (Phoenix Press, St. Louis 1984).
28 Trefler, E.: Seating for children with cerebral palsy (Univ. Tenn. Rehab. Eng. Prog., Memphis 1984).
29 Musselwhite, W.; St. Louis, K.: Communication programming for persons with severe handicaps (Little, Brown, Boston 1988).
30 Goldenberg, E.; Russell, S.; Carter, C.: Computers, education and special needs (Addison-Wesley, Reading 1984).
31 Charlebois-Marois, C.: Everybody's technology: a sharing of ideas in augmentative communication (Charlecoms, Montreal 1986).
32 Beukelman, D.; Yorkston, K.; Dowden, P.: Communication augmentation. A casebook of clinical management (College-Hill Press, San Diego 1985).
33 McDonald, E.: Treating cerebral palsy – for clinicians by clinicians (PRD-ED, Austin 1987).
34 Wright, C.; Norman, M.: From toys to computers: access for the physically disabled child (Don Johnston Developmental Equipment, Waucondal 1987).
35 Brandenberg, S.; Vanderheiden, G.: Computer, control and computer access for disabled and elderly individuals. Resource Book 1: Communication aids; Resource Book 2: Switches and environmental controls; Resource Book 3: Software and hardware (Little, Brown, Boston 1987).
36 Kohn, J.: Multiply handicapped child: severe physical and mental disability; in Bleck, Nagel, Physically handicapped children; 2nd ed., pp. 363–384 (Grune & Stratton, New York 1983).
37 Bigge, J.: Teaching individuals with physical and multiple disabilities; 2nd ed. (Merrill, Columbus 1982).
38 O'Grady, R.; et al.: Vocational predictions compared with present vocational status of 60 young adults with cerebral palsy. Devl Med. Child Neur. *27:* 775–784 (1985).
39 Wehman, P.: Competitive employment: new horizons for severly disabled individuals (Brooks, Baltimore 1981).
40 Sailor, W.; et al.: Community intensive instruction; in Horner, et al., Education of learners with severe handicaps: exemplary service strategies (Brooks, Baltimore 1985).
41 Curtis, L.: Vocational placement in cerebral palsy (United Cerebral Palsy Association, New York 1951/1953).

42 Blasco, P.; Baumgartner, M.; Mathes, B.: Literature for parents of children with cerebral palsy. Devl Med. Child Neur. *25:* 642–647 (1983).
43 Bleck, E.; Nagel, D.: Literature for parents and professionals; in Physically handicapped children, a medical atlas for teachers; 2nd ed., pp. 217–253 (Grune & Stratton, New York 1982).
44 Finnie, N.: Handling the young cerebral palsied child at home; (Dutton, New York 1975).
45 Fraser, B.; Hensinger, R.: Managing physical handicaps: a practical guide for parents, care providers, and educators (Brookes, Baltimore 1983).
46 Hale, G.: The source book for the disabled (Bantam Books, New York 1981).
47 Levy, J.: The baby exercise book (Random House, New York 1975).
48 Solomons, H.; Bottke, R.: Literature for parents of children with cerebral palsy, vol. 34, pp. 6–7 (American Academy for Cerebral Palsy & Developmental Medicine, Richmond 1982).

Received: June 23, 1989

Jean G. Kohn, MD
Lecturer and Field Program Supervisor
Maternal and Child Health Program
School of Public Health
University of California, Berkeley
Earl Warren Hall
Berkeley, CA 94720 (USA)

Pediatrician 1990;17:237–243

0300–1245/90/0174–0237$2.75/0

Burns in Children and Adolescents: Initial Management as the First Step in Successful Rehabilitation

Hugo F. Carvajal

Department of Pediatrics, University of Texas Health Science Center, Houston, Tex., USA

Key Words. Burns · Children · Adolescents · Fluid resuscitation · Acute care · Rehabilitation

Abstract. Burns, the most devastating injuries known, are the second leading cause of nonvehicular accidental deaths. Approximately one-third of these deaths occur in children less than 16 years of age. In this age group, burns are the number one cause of accidental death in the home. Successful rehabilitation begins with skilled initial management.

Data accumulated by the National Burn Information Exchange (NBIE), a voluntary registry established in 1964 [1], have shown that burn accidents occur in a disproportionate high number during the first 4 years of life and that male children are affected more often than females. This age group alone accounts for 52% of all pediatric burns.

Children are burned as a direct result of their own actions in approximately 80% of the cases, as innocent bystanders in 15–20% of the cases, and as intended victims in 2–3% of the cases.

During the first 2 years of life, 95% of the burn injuries occur indoors and the etiologic agent is a hot liquid in 80% of the patients [2]. As the child gets older the proportion of indoor injuries progressively declines and scalds become less frequent. During adolescence, 60% of the injuries occur outdoors and only 20% occur as a result of scalding [3]. The depth and extent of the burn also increase as the child gets older.

Pathophysiology of the Burn Wound

Burn injuries occur when thermal energy makes contact with skin and other tissues. Tissue damage begins at temperatures of 40 °C and increases logarithmically as the temperature rises [4]. At 45 °C denaturation of tissue proteins ensues, and recovery is no longer possible. The exact mechanism by which injury develops is not entirely clear but the noxious effects of heat and the inflammatory response that follows may persist for at least 24 h postinjury [5, 6].

Tissue damage is seldom homogenous and according to Jackson three consecutive zones of significant thermal injury can be identified: (1) the zone of coagulation which represents the area having the most intimate contact with the heat source (temperature > 45 °C); (2) the zone of stasis which extends in a three-dimensional fashion away from the zone of coagulation, and (3) the zone of hyperemia which is immediately adjacent to the zone of stasis and surrounded by unaffected tissues [7].

Burn injuries are also classified according to the depth of tissue damage into the following: (1) First degree burn, where only the superficial layer of the skin is affected. Clinically this injury is characterized by pain and redness. Within a few days the epithelium peels away from the totally healed subjacent skin without residual scarring. (2) Second degree burns are subclassified into superficial and deep. Typical of the former are pain and blister formation, while the latter is characterized by a white leathery marble-like appearance. In second degree burns the dermal appendages and other skin structures are preserved and from these reepithelization can occur. Healing usually takes place within 14–17 days. Marginally viable tissue as seen in the deeper burns can heal spontaneously but only where optimal conditions for preservation of these elements can be maintained. Conversion from partial to full thickness necrosis is a common occurrence [8]. (3) Third-degree or full thickness burns are well demarcated injuries which are not associated with blister formation. These injuries can only heal from the margins and by definition require skin grafting. They have a black or brown leathery appearance and since they are devoid of nerve endings they are painless. (4) Fourth degree burns involve not only the entire thickness of the skin but subjacent structures such as subcutaneous fat, fascia, muscle, or bone, as well. In addition to grafting, reconstructive surgery often is needed for this type of injury, and severe disfigurement is a common end result.

Table 1. ABC of burn resuscitation

Airway	assure at patent airway beware of smoke inhalation intubate early
Breathing	assure adequate ventilation and oxygenation
Circulation	estimate intravascular volume deficits maintain hemodynamic balance check central and peripheral pulses, capillary refill, heart rate, blood pressure and sensorium
Depth	assess depth and if circulation is compromised perform escharotomies early
Extent	map partial and full thickness burns calculate total burned area in m^2

Table 2. Body proportions (%) according to age [modified from 10]

Body area	0–4 years	5–9 years	10–14 years
Head and neck	19	15	13
Anterior trunk	16	17	17
Posterior trunk	16	17	17
Right arm	9	9	9
Left arm	9	9	9
Right leg	15	16	17
Left leg	15	16	17

Acute Care

Successful retrieval of the burned child from the most catastrophic injury known requires a multidisciplinary approach and a carefully delineated plan of management. The latter must be known to every member of the burn team and must be rehearsed in advance of the first patient to be treated. This is particularly important when caring for infants or young children, where the margins of safety are narrower, and therapeutic errors tend to have graver consequences than in older children or adults.

Care must be administered in an orderly fashion, following the same principles of resuscitation that have been outlined for other life-threatening conditions (table 1). All unconscious patients, and those with respiratory distress suspected of smoke inhalation, must be intubated at the scene. Severe bronchospasm and progressive edema of the upper airway are common complications of smoke inhalation or inhalation of heated air or steam and must be anticipated. If cardiopulmonary resuscitation is required at the scene or additional evidence of smoke inhalation is uncovered (carbonaceous sputum, singed nasal hairs, inspiratory stridor, damage to the pharyngeal or laryngotracheal mucosa, etc.) the patient must remain intubated for 3–5 days.

Hemodynamic stability must be assessed by palpating for central and peripheral pulses, checking for capillary refill, evaluating sensorium changes and measuring blood pressure. If the patient is in shock, fluid therapy must be initiated at once. Every attempt should be made to establish an intravenous line, but if this cannot be accomplished swiftly, drug and fluid administration must be initiated by the intraosseous route. A safe rate of fluid infusion (unlikely to result in complications) is 20 ml/kg or 600 ml/m^2 of body surface over 30–60 min. This quantity can be repeated every hour, until more precise calculations can be made.

The stomach is emptied with a nasogastric tube and 30 ml/m^2 of body surface of an antacid (i.e. Maalox) is instilled to retard the development of stress ulcers [9]. A Foley catheter is inserted in the urinary bladder, the urine drained out and the time noted. The body surface area is then estimated. This requires measurements of weight and height and the use of standard nomograms (fig. 1). The wounds must be cleansed, debrided and their depth and extent mapped using body proportions corrected for age (table 2). Circumferential deep second or third degree burns are inspected and their tourniquet effect evaluated to avoid limb ischemia, and/or respira-

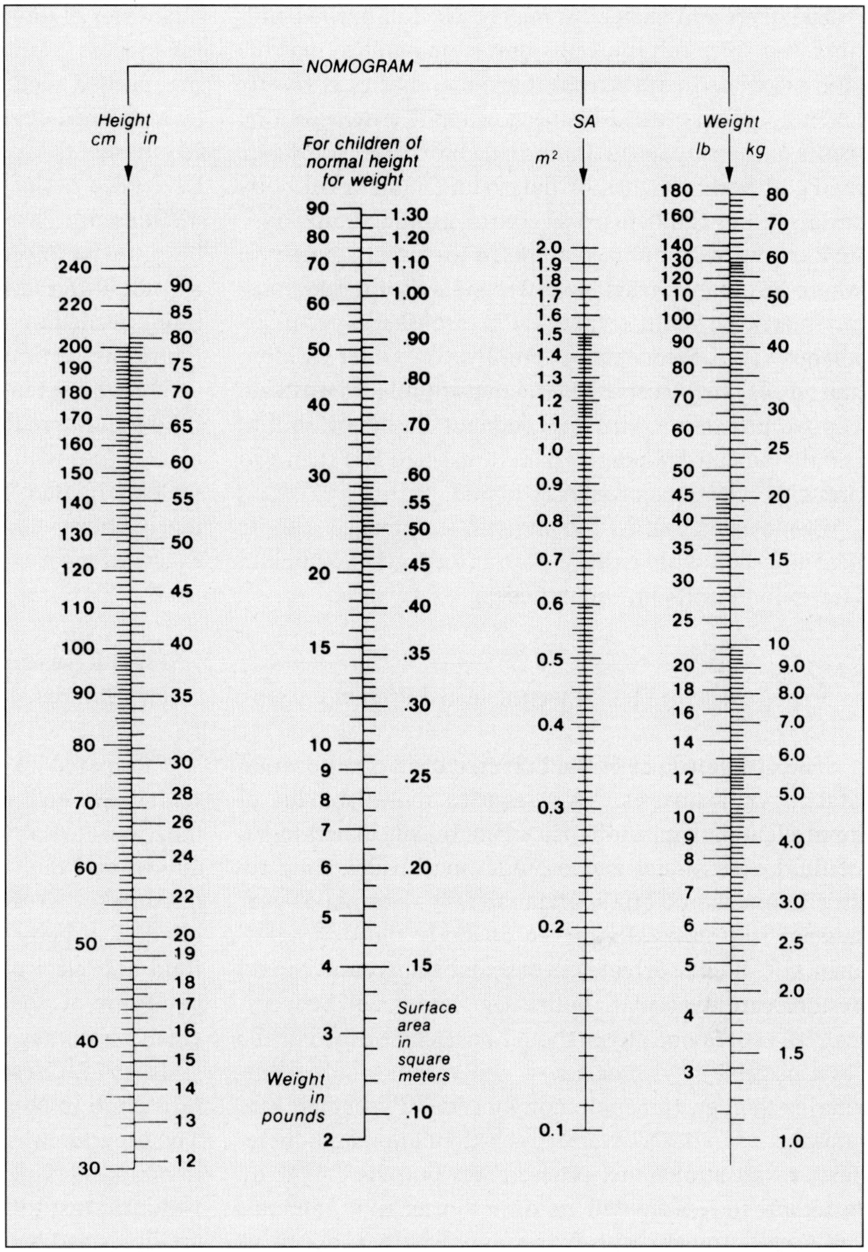

Fig. 1. Surface area nomogram. Greater accuracy can be attained by measuring height and weight and calculating body surface area by the intersect of this line [with permission, 15].

tory embarrassment resulting from chest wall involvement. Escharotomies should be performed early, before edema sets in and the circulation is further compromised [10, 11].

Once the wounds have been cleansed and debrided and, if indicated, escharotomies performed, the burns are covered with dressings saturated with an antimicrobial agent. In children, silver sulfadiazine cream continues to be the agent of choice. A 1% concentration is well above the concentration necessary to inhibit the growth of organisms in vitro, and is therefore likely to delay colonization of the wound with bacteria [12]. Silver sulfadiazine must be applied to the wounds liberally, on a daily basis, then covered with one layer of gauze and held in place with an elastic net. Except for occasional sensitivity reactions, and rarely associated leukopenia, this topical agent is well tolerated. Its low absorption through denuded skin, painless application, and low toxicity have made it the preferred topical agent in burned children [13].

Sedatives and analgesics may be used in burned children, but since full thickness burns are painless and the pain associated with partial thickness injuries is greatly ameliorated once the dressings are applied, their routine use is not mandatory. If needed, morphine (0.05–0.1 mg/kg of body weight), or diazepam (5 mg/m^2 of body surface/dose) can be used to control pain and anxiety.

Previously immunized children (0–6 years of age) in whom less than 5 years have elapsed since the last booster injection should receive DPT (diphtheria-pertussis-tetanus vaccine) for tetanus prophylaxis. Older children and adults must receive TD (tetanus-diphtheria) instead. Passive protection with TIG (tetanus immunoglobulin) is only indicated when the patient has had less than two previous injections of tetanus toxoid.

Prophylaxis against β-hemolytic streptococci can be accomplished with a single dose of benzatine penicillin (1.2 million units intramuscularly).

Replacement of Fluid, Electrolyte and Protein Losses

The ultimate goal of fluid resuscitation is restoration of body homeostasis. This requires replenishment of antecedent deficits and replacement of concurrent losses of fluid, electrolytes and protein. Specifically, fluid resuscitation should attain and maintain a normal or near normal state of hydration in all body fluid compartments; it should correct acid base imbalance, and should restore cardiovascular, pulmonary and renal hemodynamics. These objectives should be accomplished at the least possible physiologic cost and without adding further pathology (primum non nocere). Particular care must be taken not to overload the circulation and, therefore, rehydration must proceed slowly (over 24–48 h). Attempts to replace deficits over shorter time intervals are usually fraught with many complications, excessive edema and cardiopulmonary congestion.

The physician must recognize that in response to the injury a number of compensatory mechanisms are called into play and that therapeutic interventions must proceed in unison rather than oppose the organism's attempts to restore homeostasis. For example, studies in animals and humans [14–16] have shown that oliguria, a normal physiologic response to volume deficit, cannot be completely reversed by fluid replacement, and that attempts to increase urine output by excessive fluid administration may be associated with fluid retention and edema formation. Likewise, rapid restoration of cardiac output to preburn control levels requires such large quantities of fluid that the complications encountered in the process far outweigh the potential advantages of having reached such endpoint [17].

In burned children the difficulties in estimating fluid requirements are magnified, because most formulas have been designed for adult individuals and their predictions are based solely on body weight and percent burn; furthermore, the newer versions of these formulas do not differentiate between maintenance fluids and fluids needed to replace burn-related losses. Instead both figures are estimated together ('single figure formulas', i.e. 3 ml/kg/% burn, etc.). Under these circumstances, the fluid requirements of young or small children and particularly those with small burns (less than 25%) tend to be underestimated; while large or obese children with extensive burns end up receiving quantities of fluid far in excess of what is needed for successful rehydration.

Fluid Resuscitation Program Specifically Designed for Children

Compared to adults, children (and particularly infants) have high rates of heat and water exchange. Their muscle water content and composition is different from adults, and their insensible water losses and urine production are greater than in adults, when expressed in relation to body weight. Thus, in children estimates of fluid and electrolyte requirements based on energy expenditure or body surface area rather than weight offer greater accuracy, consistency and simplicity.

In 1975, Carvajal [18] developed a formula and fluid resuscitation program specifically designed for children. The program was successfully tested in humans [16] and in animals [19–21] and has since been adopted by many pediatric institutions. The key features of this program are described below.

Estimates of Total Fluid Requirements

These are based on body surface area and surface area burned and are calculated according to a pediatric burn formula: 5,000 ml/m^2 of body surface *burned*/24 h (burn-related losses), and 2,000 ml/m^2 of total body surface/24 h (maintenance fluids).

Half of the 24-hour fluid allowance is given during the first 8 h and the other half during the subsequent 16 h (fig. 2). No ceiling for burn size is used, and all fluids are administered intravenously at a relatively constant rate. Except for Maalox (30 ml/m^2 of body surface/h) the patient is kept NPO.

Composition of the Hydrating Solution

The fluid resuscitation program uses only one hydrating solution (composite solution), which can be prepared by mixing 50 ml of 25% human serum albumin (12.5 g) with 950 ml of 5% dextrose in lactated Ringer's injection. The final electrolyte and protein concentration of this solution is: Na^+ 132.0 mEq/l, Cl^- 109.0 mEq/l, lactate 26.6 mEq/l, K^+ 3.8 mEq/l, glucose 47.5 g/l, and albumin 12.5 g/l.

In infants less than 12 months of age, isotonic salt solutions may result in hypernatremia. Therefore, a modified solution has been proposed for children less than 1 year of age. This can be prepared by mixing 930 ml of 5% dextrose and 0.33% sodium chloride injection, 20 ml of sodium bicarbonate injection (1 mEq/ml) and 50 ml of 25% human serum albumin. The final composition of this solution for infants is: Na^+ 81 mEq/l, Cl^- 61 mEq/l, HCO_3^- 20 mEq/l, K^+ 0, glucose 46.5 g/l, and albumin 12.5 g/l.

Potassium replacement should not be attempted until the young patient's rehydration is well underway and normal kidney function has been ascertained. This seldom occurs before 16–24 h after the burn, at which point 20–30 mEq/l of potassium phosphate may be added to the resuscitation fluids.

The major advantage of using a composite solution is that fluid and electrolytes and protein are replaced simultaneously in quantities that approximate the losses and therefore only the rate of infusion may need adjustment.

Guidelines to Fluid Resuscitation

Choosing the proper guideline to monitor the results of therapy and clearly defining the endpoint of the fluid resuscitation effort are essential prerequisites of a successful resuscitation program. Furthermore, since no single criterion can be used to predict the state of hydration reliably and consistently, as many indicators as possible must be correlated before a decision to alter the plan of hydration is made (table 3).

Measurement of hourly urine output should be discouraged as marked fluctuations in urine production are the rule rather than the exception. This is because a state of antidiuresis, similar to the syndrome of inappropriate secretion or antidiuretic hormone, usually develops in response to the burn trauma and secretion of the hormone does not seem to correlate with intravascular volume deficit or excess. This plus an increase in vascular permeability sets the stage for accumulation of large quantities of fluids in the interstitial space (burn edema) and as a consequence, blood flow to distal areas is compromised.

Human and animal studies have shown that the hourly urine output varies greatly despite constant fluid administration [15]. This may be due to intermittent secretion of ADH, rapid degradation of the hormone and/or reflex-mediated changes in renal hemodynamics. Whatever the cause, this variable is unreliable to guide hydration and should not be used to substantiate the need for fluid pushes.

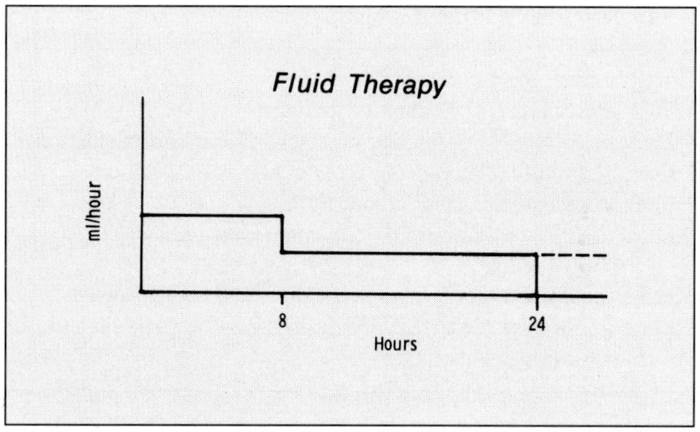

Fig. 2. Schematic representation of fluid administration during the first 24 h postinjury.

Table 3. Hydration guides

Physical exam	general appearance vital signs sensorium venous capillary filling weight
Laboratory	HCT BUN electrolytes and osmolality (serum and urine) ABGs
Fluid losses	urine ouput[1] gastrointestinal losses
Invasive monitoring[2]	cardiac output wedge pressure oxygen consumption oxygen extraction

1 Marked fluctuations in urine output (15–45 ml/m^2/h) are the rule.
2 Rarely necessary.

Table 4. Pitfalls of fluid resuscitation

Errors in measuring body surface area
Errors in estimating the extent of the burn
Failure to correct for deficits of excesses in fluid administration
Failue to correct for oliguria in cases of acute renal failure
Failure to recognize a state of antidiuresis
Failure to adjust sodium intake for infants less than 12 months of age
Failure to adjust fluids in patients with smoke inhalation
Failure to estimate the extent of tissue damage in patients with electrical injuries

While none of the variables listed in table 3 are consistently accurate by themselves, when correlated as a group and when trends instead of individual measurements are used, the state of hydration can be more precisely assessed. For example, a conscious and alert child who follows commands is usually well hydrated. The lethargic, thirsty and anxious patient, with decreased capillary filling and/or evidence of peripheral vascular insufficiency (cold, dry, discolored and mottled skin) is obviously dehydrated. A rapid thready pulse and a high respiratory rate would also be indicative of volume contraction.

The dehydrated patient usually presents with a high hematocrit (hemoconcentration) and as the intravascular volume is restored, the hematocrit progressively declines. Failure to demonstrate this change would be indicative of persistent volume deficit. Certain variables can also be misleading. For example, a rising specific gravity or urine osmolarity are indicative of ADH secretion, but not necessarily volume contraction. If present the latter can be confirmed by also demonstrating a decreased urinary sodium (<20 mEq/l).

In general, agreement between the amount of fluids predicted by the surface area formula and the actual fluid required for successful resuscitation has been excellent, and major discrepancies have only occurred as a result of errors. The most common of these discrepancies are listed in table 4. For additional information the reader is referred to more extensive reviews [22].

Second and Subsequent Days

After the first 24 h and once the capillary permeability has been restored, fluid losses resulting from the injury occur primarily in the form of burn exudate and evaporation through denuded skin. Thus, during the second and subsequent days fluid requirements may be estimated as follows: 3,750 ml/m^2 of body surface *burned*/day (burn-related losses) and 1,500 ml/m^2 of total body surface/day (maintenance fluids).

Fluids may be administered intravenously or orally and must contain 50 mEq of sodium/l to satisfy the increased sodium losses that these patients experience in the form of burn exudate.

Potassium requirements after the 2nd day are satisfied by administering solutions containing potassium in concentrations of 30–40 mEq/l. The phosphate rather than the chloride form is preferred to simultaneously replace phosphate losses which can be considerable in burned patients.

Nutritional Requirements

The hypermetabolism associated with burn injury generally subsides when the majority of the burns are grafted or healed. Until then aggressive nutritional support is essential to prevent the consequences of malnutrition. Caloric requirements are best estimated on the basis of body surface area [23] as follows: 2,200 kcal/m^2 of body surface *burned*/day (burn-related needs) and 1,800 kcal/m^2 of total body surface/day (maintenance requirements).

In a study of 52 severely burned children, Hildreth and Carvajal [23] demonstrated that adherence to this formula resulted in an average weight gain of 6% ($n = 40$) while those children with insufficient caloric intake ($n = 12$) lost weight.

Every effort should be made to minimize energy demands by reducing external stresses such as pain, anxiety, fear and cold which stimulate the release of catecholamines and raise energy requirements. Thus, analgesics, sedatives and external heating devices should be used liberally.

Cow's milk, or in the case of infants a comparable substitute (infant formula), represent ideal sources of calories and are generally well tolerated. Milk can be given orally or via enteral tubes and requires few additives (sodium to increase its concentration to 50 mEq/l, vitamins and trace minerals). It can provide up to 80% of the caloric needs of the patient.

Rehabilitation

More cripling diseases occur each year as a result of burn injury than at the height of the polio epidemic. Thus, the reason the term 'silent epidemic' is often used to describe the catastrophic effects of thermal injuries. Physical and psychological effects must be addressed independently and therapy should be extended beyond the child himself to include the family unit. Residual deformities and loss of function greatly impair the child's body image and self-esteem and prolonged hospitalization leads to a dependency reaction which often extends beyond the period of confinement.

Guilt feelings on the part of the child and family members must be discussed early, openly and preferably as a group. Discharge planning should be initiated at the beginning of hospitalization. The major challenge is reintegration of the child into society (home life, family, school, and other activities) in as painless manner as possible. Return to school should be encouraged within a week or two of discharge from the hospital.

Both parents and child should be instructed in home care procedures such as dressing changes, splints, pressure dressings and physical therapy. The risks of hypertrophic scar formation, contractures and other secondary deformities must be explained thoroughly and repeatedly using photographs and other visual aids. Physical and occupational therapists must maintain close ties with the child and family, and surgeons and pediatricians must support their role and efforts.

The services of mental health professionals and social workers are needed not only during the acute hospitalization but also during convalescence and in some instances for several years thereafter. The care of burn injuries requires a multidisciplinary approach. This is particularly true during the rehabilitation phase where the cooperative efforts of many health care professionals working as a team are essential to a successful outcome.

References

1 Feller, I.: Burn epidemiology: focus on youngsters and the aged. Burn Care Rehabil. *3:* 285 (1982).
2 Feller, I.: Prevention of burns in 1 and 2 year olds. NBIE Newslett., vol. 1, No. 2 (1980).
3 Green, A.: Epidemiology of burns in childhood. Burns incl. Therm. Inj. *10:* 368–371 (1984).
4 Moritz, A.; Henrique, F.: Studies of thermal injury. The relative importance of time and surface temperature in the causation of cutaneous burns. Am. J. Path. *23:* 695–920 (1947).
5 Ham, K.; Hurley, J.: An electron microscope study of the vascular response to mild thermal injury in the rat. J. Path. Bact. *95:* 175–183 (1968).
6 Branemark, P.; Breine, U.; Joshi, J.: Part I. Pathophysiology of the thermal burns. Microvascular pathophysiology of burn tissue. Ann. N.Y. Acad. Sci. *150:* 474 (1968).
7 Jackson, D.: The diagnosis of the depth of burning. Br. J. Surg. *40:* 588 (1953).
8 Order, S.; Moncrief, J.: The burn wound (Thomas, Springfield 1965).
9 Watson, L.C.; Abston, S.: Prevention of upper gastrointestinal hemorrhage in 582 burned children. Am. J. Surg. *132:* 790–795 (1976).
10 Lung, C.; Brouder, N.: The estimation of areas of burns. Surgery Gynec. Obstet. *79:* 352–358 (1944).
11 Zuker, R.: Initial management of the burn wound; in Carvajal, Parks, Burns in children, pp. 99–105 (Yearbook Medical Publishers, Chicago 1988).
12 Monafo, W.; Avyazaian, V.: Topical therapy. Surg. Clins N. Am. *58:* 1157–1171 (1978).
13 Wachtel, T.: Topical antimicrobials; in Carvajal, Parks, Burns in children, pp. 106–118 (Yearbook Medical Publishers, Chicago 1988).
14 Carvajal, H.: The optimal composition of burned resuscitation fluids. Crit. Care Med. *16:* 695–699 (1988).
15 Carvajal, H.: Controversies in fluid resuscitation; in Carvajal, Parks, Burns in children, pp. 51–77 (Yearbook Medical Publishers, Chicago 1988).
16 Carvajal, H.: A physiologic approach to fluid therapy in severely burned children. Surgery Gynec. Obstet. *150:* 379–384 (1980).
17 Pruitt, B.: Fluid resuscitation of burn patients: does clinical 'success' necessitate 'excess'? Sth. med. J. *69:* 1399 (1976).
18 Carvajal, H.: Acute management of burns in children. Sth. med. J. *68:* 129–131 (1975).
19 Carvajal, H.: Effect of burn depth upon edema formation and albumin extravasation in rats. Burns *7:* 79–83 (1980).
20 Carvajal, H.; Linares, H.: Relationship of burn size to vascular permeability changes in rats. Surgery Gynec. Obstet. *149:* 193–202 (1979).
21 Carvajal, H.; Reinhard, J.; Traber, D.: Renal and cardiovascular functional response to thermal injury in dogs subjected to sympathetic blockade. Circulation Shock *3:* 287–298 (1976).
22 Carvajal, H.; Parks, D.: Burns in children (Yearbook Medical Publishers, Chicago 1988).
23 Hildreth, M.; Carvajal, H.: Caloric requirements in burned children: a simple formula to estimate daily caloric requirements. J. Burn Care Rehabil. *3:* 78–80 (1982).

Received: July 7, 1989

H.F. Carvajal, MD
Professor of Pediatrics and Surgery
Department of Pediatrics
University of Texas Health Science Center
Houston, TX 77030 (USA)

Pediatrician 1990;17:244–254

0300–1245/90/0174–0244$2.75/0

Pediatric Spinal Cord Injury: Treatment and Outcome

Teresa L. Massagli[a], *Kenneth M. Jaffe*[a, b]

Departments of [a]Rehabilitation Medicine, and [b]Pediatrics and Neurological Surgery, University of Washington School of Medicine, Children's Hospital and Medical Center, Seattle, Wash., USA

Key Words. Spinal cord injury · Rehabilitation

Abstract. Spinal cord injury results in dramatic disturbances of motor, sensory and autonomic function. Every aspect of a child's life is significantly and usually irreversibly altered. As a condition with low incidence and protean manifestations, the acute care and rehabilitation of spinal cord injured children requires the specialized care, knowledge and experience of a multidisciplinary team found in regional centers. Functional outcome depends on the level and completeness of the spinal cord injury, comprehensive training and education, and the skillful prescription of adaptive technology and aids. Long-term care and management by rehabilitation personnel in concert with the primary care pediatrician will ensure the maintenance of functional independence and general health.

The treatment of spinal cord injury (SCI) and its resultant motor, sensory and autonomic dysfunction has improved dramatically in the last 50 years. Although repair of the damaged neurons is still impossible, advances in medical management and technology have had a significant impact on morbidity, mortality and quality of life in these patients. The purpose of this paper is to familiarize health care professionals with the care and rehabilitation of children with spinal cord injury.

Etiology and Epidemiology

The incidence of acute SCI in the United States is estimated to be 28–50 injuries/million/year, with a prevalence of over 200,000 cases [1]. Although two-thirds of cases occur in persons under age 30 years, less than 5% of all spinal cord injuries occur in children under age 16 [2].

The most common cause of SCI in all age groups is trauma. For children, motor vehicle accidents (41.5%) are the leading etiology followed by sports (27%), violence (20.5%) and falls (9.4%). Two-thirds of sports-related SCI are due to diving accidents. Other causes include football, skiing, sledding, surfing, trampoline, wrestling, gymnastics and horseback riding. Traumatic SCI occurs more frequently in boys, during the summer months, and on weekends. Quadriplegia (injury between the first cervical and the first thoracic nerve roots) accounts for 56% of the cases of SCI and paraplegia (injury below the first thoracic nerve roots) for 44% [2].

In children, relatively minor trauma can be responsible for serious myelopathy (damage or disease of the spinal cord), especially of the cervical cord [3, 4]. The anatomy and biomechanics of the immature cervical spine differ significantly from that of the adult. Children have greater mobility of the cervical spine due to ligamentous laxity, shallow angulation of the facet joints, incomplete ossification of the vertebral bodies and relative underdevelopment of neck muscles for the size of the head [5]. Because of these features, cervical SCI in the younger child is more common at the upper cervical levels than in adults [6], and often occurs in the absence of radiographic abnormality [4].

Neonatal SCI can result from forceful traction and angulation of the spine during delivery. Extradural hematoma or direct cord damage including transection can occur. Usually the fetus is delivered with a hyperextended head from either a transverse lie or breech presentation. The most frequent level of neonatal SCI is at the cervicothoracic junction; these infants have a better chance of survival than those with higher lesions. Electromyography and somatosensory-evoked potentials may be useful in differentiating neonatal SCI from primary neuromuscular disease or asphyxia [7–9].

Certain disorders carry an increased risk of injury to the cervical spinal cord. Atlantoaxial instability occurs in 10–20% of children with Down syndrome, but only 1–2% of these children develop myelopathy [10, 11]. Atlantoaxial instability and myelopathy have also been reported in juvenile rheumatoid arthritis [12]. Dysplasia of the base of the skull or cervical vertebrae can result in cervicomedullary compression in children with achondroplasia and other skeletal dysplasias [13, 14].

Nontraumatic causes of SCI include tumor, transverse myelitis, epidural abscess, and arteriovenous malformation. The onset can be insidious leading to a delayed or erroneous diagnosis. Intra- or extramedullary spinal cord tumors occur most commonly in the thoracic cord. The prognosis depends on age, the type, location and resectability of the tumor, spine stability, and the dose of radiation to the spinal cord [15]. Epidural abscess can result from hematogenous spread of osteomyelitis, or skin and soft tissue infections. *Staphylococcus aureus* is the most common organism [16]. Epidural abscess and viral-related transverse myelopathy usually affect the thoracic cord [16, 17]. Rarely, multiple sclerosis presents as myelopathy in childhood [18]. Arteriovenous malformations of the spinal cord are usually asymptomatic during childhood. They occur most often in the thoracic cord, and can be associated with bony anomalies of the vertebrae, congenital heart disease, and cutaneous angiomas [19].

Due to the low incidence of nontraumatic SCI, survival data are available only for traumatic injuries. For children under age 19 years who survive to be discharged from the hospital, 10-year survival is estimated at 90–93% [2]. With proper medical care a normal life expectancy can be anticipated [20].

It has been recommended recently that SCI should become the first injury condition reportable to state health agencies and the Centers for Disease Control [1]. This surveillance would more accurately determine the incidence and causes of traumatic SCI, identify high-risk groups, and guide the development of prevention programs. Pediatric health professionals have an important role in identifying children at risk for injury and in educating families regarding proper seat belt and helmet use, household safety, behavioral risks and environmental hazards [21].

Initial Management

In most cases of SCI, the cord is damaged by blunt, nonpenetrating injury and is not lacerated or transected. It is thus imperative to avoid injudicious management which may produce further injury and disability. SCI and spine instability should always be suspected in the unconscious trauma victim. The conscious child should be questioned regarding neck or back pain and examined for sensory or motor disturbance. At the scene of the injury, it is important to immobilize the spine for transport, assess for life-threatening signs, and protect the airway [22]. The child should be placed on a spinal board with neck rotation prevented by sandbags. All hard objects must be removed from clothing to prevent pressure sores. In the young child, positioning on the standard backboard may produce relative cervical kyphosis due to the size of the head compared to the body. An occipital cut-out to lower the head or a mattress to raise the body should be used to horizontally align the external auditory meatus with the shoulder [23].

At the hospital, spine stability must be maintained during subsequent examinations and procedures, and skin pressure relief must be provided at least every 1–2 h. A thorough physical examination is undertaken to search for associated trauma, especially to the head, chest and extremities [2]. Signs of intraabdominal injury can be masked in patients with SCI above the seventh thoracic level [24]. A Foley catheter is inserted because the bladder is initially noncontractile. Paralytic ileus often ensues after severe SCI and a nasogastric tube may be needed. In the severly brain-injured or unconscious child, the diagnosis of SCI can be very difficult. Clues include a dermatomal pattern of sensory loss, symmetric absence of reflexes, flaccidity, absence of sacral reflexes, unexplained urinary retention or ileus, or priapism [25].

Neurologic Exam

A careful neurologic exam will define the motor and sensory level and the completeness of the SCI. Muscle strength is commonly graded as 0 (no contraction), 1 or trace (feeble contraction), 2 or poor (full active movement in a gravity-eliminated position), 3 or fair (ability to move and hold in an antigravity position), 4 or good (able to take some resistance) and 5 or normal (able to

Table 1. Key reflexes and muscles

Nerve root	Reflexes	Muscles and function
C4		diaphragm: inspiration
C5	biceps (C5, C6)	deltoid: shoulder flexion and abduction
		biceps: elbow flexion
C6		extensor carpi radialis: wrist extension
C7	triceps (C7, C8)	triceps: elbow extension
C8		flexor digitorum superficialis: finger flexion
T1		interossei: finger abduction and adduction
T2–T7		intercostals: expiration, forced inspiration
T8–T12	superficial abdominals	abdominals: expiration, trunk flexion
L2	cremasteric (L1, L2)	iliopsoas: hip flexion
L3	knee (L3, L4)	quadriceps: knee extension
L4		tibialis anterior: foot dorsiflexion
L5	hamstring (L5, S1)	extensor hallucis longus: great toe extension
S1	ankle (S1, S2)	gastrocnemius: foot plantar flexion
S2–S4	anal wink, bulbocavernosus	anal sphincter: fecal continence

resist maximum pressure) [26]. The American Spinal Injury Association defines the SCI motor level as the lowest segment in which muscle strength is grade 3 or greater [27]. Key muscles for determination of motor level are shown in table 1. All muscles have innervation from more than one root level. Thus, if the key muscle has at least grade 3 strength, the corresponding neurologic root level should be essentially normal. The sensory level is described according to the lowest dermatome in which sensation is normal. Pinprick, light touch and proprioception are assessed to determine the integrity of the spinothalamic tracts and posterior columns. In thoracic SCI, if the umbilicus deviates superiorly on contraction of the abdominal musculature, relative weakness below T10 is present. However, the precise level of thoracic SCI is commonly assigned according to the sensory level. Complete SCI denotes no preservation of motor and/or sensory function below three root levels from the last normal level [27].

Patterns of incomplete cord injury include anterior cord syndrome with motor paralysis, reduced pain and temperature sensation, and preserved dorsal column function; central cord syndrome with flaccid weakness of the arms and relatively strong but spastic leg function, preserved sacral sensation, and preserved bladder and bowel function; posterior cord syndrome with loss of proprioception; and Brown-Séquard syndrome with homolateral paralysis and contralateral pain and temperature loss.

After SCI, there is an initial period of spinal shock. The patient is flaccid below the level of the lesion and all cutaneous and deep tendon reflexes are absent. This lasts for hours to weeks, and its end is heralded by a return of sacral reflexes; i.e., the bulbocavernosus reflex and anal wink. Injury below the L1 vertebral level can damage the conus medullaris or the cauda equina, producing a lower motor neuron injury, in which the sacral reflexes will remain permanently absent unless neurologic recovery occurs.

Determination of the level and completeness of the SCI and the presence or absence of spinal shock allows for a prognosis to be made at 24–48 h after injury [2, 5, 24, 28]. In patients with complete loss of motor and sensory function there is a slight chance of further recovery if the bulbocavernosus reflex has not returned. Anterior cord syndrome has a poor prognosis for return of function due to damage to the anterior spinal artery. In posterior cord syndrome, motor power and pain and temperature sensation can be present, but the profound loss of proprioception renders walking very difficult. In the Brown-Séquard and central cord syndromes, there is a good prognosis for walking and bladder and bowel control, but hand function usually remains impaired in the latter. Lesions of the cauda equina may show recovery over 6–24 months as neurapraxia resolves and lower motor neuron regeneration to proximal muscles occurs. Although considerable research efforts are devoted to developing physical, pharmacological and surgical approaches to the treatment of SCI, none is capable of reversing severe spinal cord damage [29].

Initial Evaluation of SCI

Following initial evaluation and stabilization of the patient, plain radiologic investigation of the spine is undertaken to diagnose bony vertebral injury such as a burst, compression or Chance fracture (a horizontal fracture through a lumbar disc or vertebra, classically due to a lap seatbelt injury), facet subluxation or dislocation. While maintaining spine stability, radiographs of the entire spine, including odontoid views, are obtained. Oblique views may be needed to confirm facet subluxations or dislocations. Myelography is rarely performed because it requires turning the patient in different positions. However, computerized axial tomography is frequently used to identify root impingement and bone fragments within the spinal canal [30]. Because severe SCI without radiographic abnormality commonly occurs in children, physical examination remains the cornerstone of diagnosis.

If spinal alignment can be restored with traction and maintained by an orthosis, surgery may not be necessary. Indications for surgery include a penetrating wound (i.e. knife or bullet), failure of closed reduction, nerve root impingement, and bone fragments compressing the cauda equina. Bone grafting and internal fixation may be necessary to maintain stability of the vertebral column and to facilitate rapid remobilization of the patient. During surgery, avoid using succinylcholine or other depolarizing agents which, in the face of denervation, can produce severe hyperkalemia leading to cardiac arrest [31]. Postoperatively, patients must wear an external orthosis until bony fusion is complete, usually for around 3 months. The long-term goals of spine management, regardless of treatment, are prevention of deformity, pain and further neurologic loss [32, 33].

Rehabilitation

Ideally, rehabilitation personnel act as consultants to the acute care team regarding the management of neurogenic bladder and blowel and the prevention of pressure sores and contractures. The provision of patient and family education, counseling and support during the acute care phase will also facilitate a smooth transition to the rehabilitation setting.

When the vertebral injury is stable, the child can be transferred to a facility or unit specializing in rehabilitation where comprehensive, multidisciplinary care is provided in a cost-effective, efficient manner [34]. The rehabilitation team typically consists of a pediatric physiatrist, rehabilitation nurses, a dietitian, occupational, physical, speech/language and recreational therapists, a social worker, a clinical psychologist, an orthotist and a teacher. The aim of rehabilitative management is to achieve the maximum independence of function within the limits imposed by the level and completeness of the SCI (see tables 2, 3). Based on these expectations and on principles of normal physical, motor, and cognitive development, appropriate short- and long-term goals are developed by the child, family and team.

Children with high quadriplegia (injury at C4 or above) pose a particular challenge. Damage to the cervical cord between C3 and C5 can produce phrenic nerve dysfunction and ventilator dependence. Patients with higher injury (brainstem to C2) have paralyzed diaphragms but intact phrenic nerves and can be candidates for implantation of phrenic nerve pacemakers [35]. Currently, most ventilator-dependent quadriplegic children are managed with a tracheostomy and positive pressure ventilation. Older teenagers can use a daytime pneumobelt (a corset-type expiration assist) [36]. An uncuffed tracheostomy tube facilitates verbal communication, but adapted talking tubes are available if cuff deflation is not possible [37]. Technologic advances allow for long-term survival and some independent function in these children [38]. They may be able to eat using a mechanical feeder and control a power wheelchair, access computers, and utilize environmental control units with chin or breath-controlled switches. With a mouthstick, participation in many educational and recreational activities is also possible. Twenty-four-hour nursing care, family training, and adaptive equipment permit a successful return to home and school [39, 40].

Greater levels of independence in self-care, mobility and communication can be expected at successively lower SCI levels (see table 2). At any given level, children with incomplete lesions have the potential for greater function than those with complete lesions. In adults, the highest level compatible with a completely independent life is C7. Children with much lower levels of injury, however, commonly require assistance with self-care activities and mobility.

Self-Care

During inpatient rehabilitation, children work with the occupational therapist and nursing staff on self-care skills such as feeding, dressing, grooming, bathing and toileting. Some need to use adaptive equipment such as built-up utensil handles, hand or wrist splints, long flexible straws or scoop dishes for feeding; dressing sticks, sock loops, zipper loops, button hooks, or velcro closures for dressing; adapted mirrors, toothpaste and deodorant dispensers for grooming; and wash mitts, tub benches, hand-held showering devices, shower chairs or long-handled sponges for bathing. Older children also work on higher level skills such as bedmaking, food preparation and other situationally and age-appropriate chores.

Neurogenic Bladder and Bowel

Patient age and SCI level also influence bowel and bladder management. Injuries which directly damage the sacral roots (S2,3,4) produce lower motor neuron dys-

Table 2. Optimal function in motor complete quadriplegia

Function	C1–C4	C5	C6	C7, C8, T1
Self-care				
Eating	dependent; drinks with long straw; can use mechanical feeder	independent using balanced forearm orthoses, splints, and adapted utensils after setup	independent with splints and adapted utensils	independent
Bathing	dependent	dependent	independent with equipment	independent
Grooming	dependent	some facial grooming possible with equipment	independent with equipment	independent
Dressing	dependent	partial assistance for upper extremities; dependent for lower extremities	independent for upper extremities; assistance for lower extremities	independent with adaptations to clothing
Toileting	dependent	dependent	independent with bowel management; assistance for bladder management	independent
Pressure relief	dependent in bed and manual wheelchair; independent with power recline wheelchair	as for C1–C4	independent	independent
Communication				
Reading	needs page turner or mouthstick	as for C1–C4	independent	independent
Writing	unable	as for C1–C4	needs hand splint	independent
Typing (electric typewriter or computer)	access with mouth or breath control or voice activation	as for C1–C4	needs hand splint	independent
Telephone	using environmental control unit, can operate phone and other appliances	as for C1–C4	independent	independent
Mobility				
Bed	dependent	assistance, even with electric bed	independent with equipment; electric bed helpful	independent; electric bed helpful
Transfers	dependent	dependent	independent with sliding board	independent; may need sliding board
Wheelchair	independent with power wheelchair with chin or mouth control	independent with power wheelchair with hand control	independent with manual wheelchair with adapted rims; assistance outdoors	independent with manual wheelchair
Transportation	unable to drive; travel by accessible van with lift	unable to drive (new technology may permit driving using joystick control); travel by accessible van with lift	independent driving with hand controls; assistance to load wheelchair into car	independent driving with hand controls; independent in loading wheelchair into car

Table 3. Optimal mobility in motor complete paraplegia

Mobility	T2–T10	T11–L2	L3–S2
Manual wheelchair	independent indoors and in community	independent indoors and in community	may not need wheelchair except for long distances (or recreation)
Ambulation	exercise only; needs long leg braces and forearm crutches or walker; not really practical for T2–T6; needs at least standby assistance	indoor ambulation with long leg braces and forearm crutches possible; some can climb stairs with railing	indoor and community ambulator with short leg braces and forearm crutches or canes; prolonged standing may be difficult
Driving	needs hand controls; independent in loading wheelchair into car	needs hand controls; independent in loading wheelchair into car	can drive automatic transmission although hand controls may be preferred

function leading to flaccid rectal and external urethral sphincters and bladder detrusor. Stool is expelled by valsalva and manual removal. Urine can also be expelled by valsalva in older children, or credé in younger ones. Flaccid sphincters predispose to incontinence with increased intraabdominal pressure (coughing or strenuous activity). Therefore, regular toileting to keep the rectum and bladder empty is essential. If necessary, α-agonist medications such as ephedrine can 'tighten' the urethral sphincter. Mature children may be candidates for an implanted artificial urinary sphincter [41].

SCI above the conus medullaris results in upper motor neuron dysfunction of the sacral segments. This causes spastic contraction of the external sphincter which diminishes the leakage of stool, but predisposes to incomplete emptying. Insertion of a gloved finger into the rectum with digital stimulation can be used to initiate a reflex evacuation. This can be supplemented with use of a glycerine or bisacodyl suppository. With a reasonable intake of fiber and fluid, patients can usually be weaned from stool softeners and bulking agents. A bedpan should not be used due to the risk of pressure-induced trauma to insensate skin.

The upper motor neuron or reflex bladder develops spontaneous contractions of the detrusor as the bladder fills. When the force of contraction exceeds the pressure generated by the internal and external sphincters, voiding results. If the external sphincter reflexly contracts simultaneously with the detrusor (detrusor-sphincter dyssynergia), inefficient emptying results. High pressures can then be generated within the bladder, predisposing to vesicoureteral reflux and bladder trabeculation. Urologic consultation and urodynamic studies can help to clarify the neurogenic bladder dysfunction. The overall goals of management are adequate emptying of the bladder, continence, and prevention of infection and upper tract damage. Quadriplegic and paraplegic children with reflex bladders are treated with anticholinergics such as oxybutinin or propantheline and intermittent catheterization. Children as young as 5 years of age can be taught self-intermittent catheterization [42]. In younger or quadriplegic children with inadequate hand function, family members can be trained to do this procedure. Sterile precautions are maintained during the hospitalization, but clean technique is substituted at home [43]. The frequency of catheterization depends on the size of the bladder and the fluid intake. Bladder capacity can be estimated as: bladder capacity (ounces) = age (years) + 2 [44]. It is reasonable to restrict fluid intake so that only four to six catheterizations per day are needed. Older males may be able to use an external collection system (condom catheter) if no dyssynergia or outlet obstruction is present. With dyssynergia, a sphincterotomy eliminates bladder outlet resistance but necessitates the use of an external collection system. Unfortunately, condom catheters do not stay on younger boys well, and no practical system of external collection has been invented for females.

Mobility

The concept of mobility is broken down into its component parts when goals are set during rehabilitation. Mobility skills include turning in bed; coming to sit; sitting balance; transferring between wheelchair, bed, toilet or car; wheelchair use (manual or power); pressure relief; ambulation; community travel and driving. The ultimate level of function is influenced by the level of impairment and residual strength, the environment and the availability of assistive technology. Tables 2 and 3 provide an overview of the optimal independence in mobility at different SCI levels.

The formulation of a wheelchair prescription requires consultation among physician, therapists, vendor, patient and family. Technologic advances and a free market system combine to present a myriad of options. The prescription must be individualized to consider patient factors such as age, growth potential, injury level, contractures, and scoliosis, and environmental factors including home architecture and outdoor terrain. Above C6, quadriplegics will need both power and manual wheelchairs. A single source of mobility is unrealistic and inadequate. A manual wheelchair provides passive mobility when the power wheelchair is broken (a common occurrence) or cannot be transported. Foam, air cell or gel cushions are commonly used to distribute pressure and stabilize the pelvis on the seat.

Ambulation is possible for paraplegics, but at any level of injury it requires increased energy expenditure [45]. Above T11, ambulation with long leg braces and assistive devices is quite slow and best viewed as exercise. At T11-L2, children need the same bracing and assistive devices, but because of better trunk and pelvic control, they can become functional indoor ambulators. Community ambulation is possible for those with adequate knee extension (L3 or below), but a manual wheelchair is still prescribed for travel over longer distances.

Driving is possible for injuries below C5, and new technology will soon allow C5 quadriplegics to drive using joystick control [46]. Spinal cord-injured adolescents of driving age are referred to a disabled driver training program to learn the use of the necessary adaptive equipment.

Functional Electrical Stimulation

Computer-assisted electrical stimulation of paralyzed skeletal muscles is now possible. Stimulation can be used to exercise leg muscles and to produce synchronized motion for ambulation. In an exercise training program, muscle bulk, strength and endurance can be increased. Significant aerobic training can be attained, but it is no greater than that achieved by maximal voluntary upper extremity activities [47]. Ambulation by electrical stimulation is possible and more successful in patients with incomplete lesions in whom only a limited number of muscles need to be stimulated. Ambulation is slow and requires bracing and upper extremity-assistive devices. At present, this research technology remains relatively unavailable and expensive [48].

Adjustment to Disability

Throughout the rehabilitation stay, the child's adjustment to disability should be carefully monitored. Adjustment can be particularly difficult for adolescents in whom the development of self-image, sexual identity and independence has been interrupted. While shock, grief and denial may be present, it is important for the child to engage in the acute rehabilitation process. If the child is participating in therapies and working toward goals, brooding over lost function is likely to diminish. A behavioral program using structure, consistency and positive reinforcement is usually successful, but some children require individual psychotherapy. Support should also be available to family members as they learn to assimilate the disability and its implications.

Sexuality and Fertility

Information about sexuality and reproductive potential is provided to families and older children. Adolescents can be assured that SCI patients remain sexually active. Females soon resume menstruation, and their fertility and ability to participate in coitus are unimpaired. Most females with complete lesions are anorgasmic but can have heightened responses to tactile stimulation above the level of the lesion. If oral contraceptive use is contemplated, progestin-only preparations are prescribed to decrease the risk of estrogen-associated deep vein thrombosis. In males, both erectile function and ejaculation are usually impaired. Reflex erections are more likely to occur in those with lesions above the sacral root level, but may be too fleeting for successful coitus. Although ejaculation occurs in some men (usually those with incomplete injuries), it is usually retrograde into the bladder. Sperm production diminishes over time, leaving very few men fertile [49]. More specific information regarding reproductive options and medical interventions can be provided as part of the long-term management.

Medical Complications

Complications occur both acutely as well as many years after SCI [50]. Prevention and early diagnosis are crucial to reducing the impact and cost of these problems.

Respiratory Complications

The diaphragm and intercostal muscles can be partially or completely paralyzed depending on the SCI level and completeness. The resultant decrease in vital capacity and forced expiration is further compromised in the upright position. Weak abdominal muscles allow the diaphragm to be pulled down by gravity, thereby restricting the diaphragmatic excursion. Due to the impaired ability to cough and clear secretions, these children are at increased risk for the development of atelectasis and pneumonia. Administration of pneumococcal and influenza vaccines should be considered. Caregivers should be taught assisted coughing techniques. Vital capacity can be increased passively, with the use of an abdominal binder when seated [51] or actively, using techniques such as glossopharyngeal or neck breathing [52]. Inspiratory muscle training can increase both the strength and endurance of the diaphragm, but has not been shown to be associated with decreased morbidity [53].

Cardiovascular Complications

Sympathetic outflow is interrupted in lesions above the midthoracic levels. Bradycardia and postural hypotension occur due to unopposed vagal tone and decreased systemic vascular resistance. Careful fluid management is warranted to avoid overinfusion and pulmonary edema. Bradycardia resolves shortly after injury, but postural hypotension can be a chronic problem. When patients are symptomatic from orthostasis, they should be reclined until the symptoms resolve. Use of elastic stockings and abdominal binders, and maintenance of hydration are useful preventive measures. Occasionally, salt supplementation or ephedrine are needed.

Deep venous thrombosis and pulmonary embolism can occur in immobilized children, especially teenagers. Phlebotomy and placement of intravenous lines in paralyzed lower extremities are contraindicated. Trauma to the vessel wall and intravenous infusions further increase the risk of deep venous thrombosis. Minidose heparinization, intermittent pneumatic compression, antiembolism stockings, and monitoring of calf and thigh circumferences are common practices in prevention and early detection [50, 54].

Neurologic Complications

Patients with complete SCI above T6 can develop autonomic hyperreflexia (dysreflexia) in which reflex sympathetic vasoconstriction occurs below the level of the SCI with secondary vasodilation above [55]. Signs and symptoms include a life-threatening, sudden rise in systolic and diastolic blood pressure, bradycardia, and a pounding headache. Sweating and flushing are present above the injury level. Triggering stimuli include bladder or bowel distention, urinary tract infection, skin wounds, or an acute abdomen. Immediate treatment is indicated to prevent complications such as hypertensive encephalopathy, seizure or cerebrovascular accident. After sitting the patient up, the triggering stimulus should be identified and removed, if possible. If this fails to reduce the blood pressure, nitropaste, sublingual nifedipine, or hydralazine can be administered. Episodes usually become less frequent over time, but can persist for years.

With lesions above the midthoracic level, loss of vasomotor control and the ability to shiver or sweat below the injury level produce impaired temperature regulation. Such patients are sensitive to changes in environmental temperature and are essentially 'poikilothermic'. Environmentally induced temperature elevation is often difficult to distinguish from other sources of fever.

Spasticity often ensues after upper motor neuron injury. It can become severe enough to cause pain, decreased range of motion, or interference with volitional control and function. It is often aggravated by infection, inflammation or state of mind. Therapeutic options include removal of aggravating stimuli, stretching exercises, and medications including baclofen, dantrolene sodium or diazepam. Chemical neurolysis and surgical ablative procedures are reserved for refractory cases [56].

A variety of pain syndromes are associated with spinal cord injury. Pain can be felt above, at, or below the lesion level. Dysesthetic pain is common, particularly after cauda equina injury. These syndromes do not respond well to opiates, but may be relieved by low doses of antidepressants such as amitriptyline or with the use of transcutaneous electrical nerve stimulation [50].

Long-term neurologic follow-up is necessary to monitor for deterioration of motor function due to spinal cord cavitation (syringomyelia). Myelography or magnetic resonance imaging are used to diagnose this problem [57].

Renal Complications

Urinary tract infection is the most common complication after SCI. Chronic infection can cause either bladder or kidney calculi and progressive loss of renal function. Depending on the lesion level, signs and symptoms can include vague abdominal discomfort, dysreflexia, increased spasticity, new onset incontinence and/or fever. Fever does not, however, help to localize the infection to either the upper or lower urinary tract. Diagnosis is confirmed by urine culture. Patients with indwelling catheters, vesicostomies, or on intermittent catheterization commonly have chronic bacterial colonization. The treatment of asymptomatic bacteriuria is controversial [58]. It probably does not decrease the incidence of febrile or symptomatic urinary tract infection. Children with symptoms, pyuria, and a positive urine culture are treated with oral antibiotics for 7–10 days. Bacteremia or pyelonephritis requires intravenous treatment [59].

Annual follow-up is necessary to monitor renal function. If suspected, calculi can be detected on plain radiographs or by ultrasound. Ultrasound or excretory urography are used for anatomic examination of the kidneys to detect reflux or scarring. Serum creatinine and creatinine clearance are insensitive measures of renal function after SCI due to the loss of muscle mass. Renal scintigraphy can be used to provide an estimate of individual kidney function [60].

Cutaneous Complications

Pressure sores, although preventable, are one of the more common and costly complications of SCI [2]. Frequently affected sites include the skin overlying the sacrum, trochanter, heel, ischium, scapula and occiput. When ulcers develop, aggressive treatment will avoid deep space infection, osteomyelitis and the need for surgery. Treatment measures include strict pressure relief, avoidance of shear forces, local wound care and debridement, and optimal nutrition. Severe wounds require surgical closure.

Gastrointestinal Complications

In the first month after SCI ileus, stress ulcers and gastric distention can occur. The most common chronic problem is fecal impaction which is avoided by regular bowel emptying. Intraabdominal emergencies are difficult to diagnose, and are associated with dysreflexia, increased spasticity, referred pain above the lesion level, change in bowel tones, and reflex abdominal guarding or spasm. Timely diagnosis requires a high index of suspicion.

Metabolic/Endocrine Complications

To prevent protein catabolism following the acute injury, a high-calorie high-protein diet is offered. Many patients experience excessive weight gain due to relative immobility and decreased basal metabolic rate. Obesity is not simply a health risk to be prevented. It also impairs the ability to transfer or ambulate.

Immobilization from any cause results in increased urinary calcium excretion within days of confinement. In SCI, hypercalciuria persists for many months, predisposing patients to urolithiasis. Unique to children, particularly adolescent boys, is immobilization hypercalcemia which usually presents 4–12 weeks after SCI [61]. Because the signs and symptoms are nonspecific (lethargy, alteration of mood, nausea, anorexia, polyuria and polydipsia), serial serum calciums should be obtained. The mainstays of treatment include remobilization, when possible, and intravenous saline infusion. Furosemide, calcitonin or etidronate can be added if necessary [62]. Restriction of dietary calcium and oral phosphate administration are ineffective.

Musculoskeletal Complications

Osteopenia (decreased bone density) develops in paralyzed extremities and increases the risk of pathologic fractures (the clinical syndrome of osteoporosis). Fractures can also occur during overaggressive range of motion exercises. Contractures result from immobilization, spasticity, and muscle imbalance across joints. They can be prevented with daily range of motion exercises and use of resting splints. Scoliosis develops in virtually all children who experience SCI prior to skeletal maturation [5]. Careful monitoring, especially during the accelerated growth spurt of puberty, is warranted. Spinal instrumentation and fusion are the only methods which successfully control progressive scoliosis.

Heterotopic ossification, the deposition of new bone in periarticular soft tissue, can affect the hips, knees, elbows and shoulders. Appearing 1–2 months after injury as local warmth, redness and swelling, this complication can result in loss of joint range of motion despite an active therapy program. It can be confused with cellulitis, septic arthritis, thrombophlebitis or fracture. Surgical removal may be necessary if bony ankylosis results in functional compromise, but should not be attempted until the bone is fully mature as determined by bone scan. Although treatment with etridronate and indomethacin have been recommended, there is no convincing evidence that either medication retards progression of the ossification [63].

Discharge Planning, Community Reentry, and Long-Term Follow-Up

Ideally, discharge planning begins upon admission to the rehabilitation program. In anticipation of permanent disability, each professional has the responsibility to make the patient and family knowledgeable in spinal injury care. To achieve the appropriate levels of training and independence, paraplegics need 1–3 months and quadriplegics 4 or more months of inpatient rehabilitation.

Skills learned in the hospital must be tested in the 'real world' of home and community, away from the direct supervision of hospital staff. Recently learned skills must be generalized to the community setting. Children and their families must become able to deal with uneven terrain, curbs, public bathrooms, transportation, and the stares of curious strangers. Passes to home provide opportunities to function away from the protective, accessible hospital environment, practice what has been learned, and identify problems and participate in their solution. Architectural barriers at home require early identification so that modifications such as ramps, widened doorways, and grab bars around the toilet or tub can be made.

Return to school is a major goal. In addition to acquiring academic or vocational skills, school is the major setting in which children develop social skills, self-esteem, work habits and expectations, and experience success and failure [64]. By meeting with school personnel prior to reentry, the rehabilitation team can provide important information regarding medical problems, bladder and bowel management, skin protection, medications, and level of independence. Realistic understanding of the child's disability enables school personnel to avoid either an inappropriately restrictive or an overly indulgent posture. Children whose disability has an impact on education can be certified as 'health-impaired'. Under federal law this enables them to receive adaptive services such as physical and occupational therapy.

Because the disabling effects of SCI are so far-reaching, discharge from the inpatient rehabilitation program should be the beginning of a comprehensive scheme for the provision of rehabilitation services to these children and families. The pediatrician continues to be the ongoing source of primary medical care. Working together with a pediatric physiatrist or other physician knowledgeable about SCI, chronic disease and disability, they strive to prevent secondary medical complications and to optimize independent functioning. Ideally, care remains community-based but is complemented by periodic follow-up visits to the rehabilitation center where evaluations by the physiatrist, nurse, and occupational and physical therapists are undertaken. Subspecialty care with a pediatric urologist and spine orthopedist is arranged as needed. Referral to a local or regional SCI society can serve as an avenue for additional support, information and advocacy.

Despite the global impact of SCI, much can be done to minimize its disabling consequences. For the pediatrician who chooses to remain involved in the care of these children, the rewards and satisfactions are sustaining.

References

1 Centers for Disease Control: Acute traumatic spinal cord injury surveillance – United States, 1987. MMWR 1988;37:285–286.
2 Stover SL, Fine PR, Go BK, et al: Spinal Cord Injury: The Facts and Figures. Birmingham, University of Alabama Press, 1986.
3 Chen LS, Blaw ME: Acute central cervical cord syndrome caused by minor trauma. J Pediatr 1986;108:96–97.
4 Pang D, Wilberger JE: Spinal cord injury without radiographic abnormalities in children. J Neurosurg 1982;57:114–129.
5 Wilberger JE: Spinal Cord Injuries in Children. New York, Futura Publ. 1986.
6 Jones ET, Hensinger RN: Cervical spine injuries in children. Comtemp Orthop 1982;5:17–23.
7 Franken EA: Spinal cord injury in the newborn infant. Pediatr Radiol 1975;3:101–104.
8 Koch BM, Eng GM: Neonatal spinal cord injury. Arch Phys Med Rehabil 1979;60:378–381.
9 Bell HJ, Dykstra DD: Somatosensory evoked potentials as an adjunct to diagnosis of neonatal spinal cord injury. J Pediatr 1985;106:298–301.
10 Committee on Sports Medicine: Atlantoaxial instability in Down syndrome. Pediatrics 1984;74:152–154.
11 Pueschel SM, Herndon JA, Gelch MM, et al: Symptomatic atlantoaxial subluxation in persons with Down syndrome. J Pediatr Orthop 1984;4:682–688.
12 Nathan FF, Bickel WH: Spontaneous axial subluxation in a child as the first sign of juvenile rheumatoid arthritis. J Bone Joint Surg 1968;50-A:1675–1678.
13 Yang SS, Corbett DP, Brough AJ, et al: Upper cervical myelopathy in achondroplasia. Am J Clin Pathol 1977;68:68–72.
14 Wynne-Davies R, Hall CM, Apley AG: Atlas of Skeletal Dysplasias. New York, Churchill Livingstone, 1985.
15 Cohen ME, Duffner PK: Tumors of the brain and spinal cord including leukemic involvement; in Swaiman KF (ed): Pediatric Neurology: Principles and Practice. St. Louis, Mosby, 1989, pp 661–714.
16 Baker AS, Ojemann RG, Swartz MN, et al: Spinal epidural abscess. N Engl J Med 1975;293:463–468.
17 Paine RS, Byer RK: Transverse myelopathy in childhood. Am J Dis Child 1953;85:151–163.
18 Schneider RD, Ong BH, Moran MJ, et al: Multiple sclerosis in early childhood. Clin Pediatr 1969;8:115–118.
19 Tobin WD, Layton DD: The diagnosis and natural history of spinal cord arteriovenous malformations. Mayo Clin Proc 1976; 51:637–646.
20 DeVivo MJ, Fine PR, Maetz HM, et al: Prevalence of spinal cord injury: A reestimation employing life table techniques. Arch Neurol 1980;37:707–708.

21 Greensher J: Recent advances in injury prevention. Pediatr Rev 1988;10:171–176.
22 Swain A, Grundy D, Russell J: ABC of spinal cord injury: At the accident. Br Med J 1985;291:1558–1560.
23 Herzenberg JE, Hensigner RN, Dedrick DK, et al: Emergency transport and positioning of young children who have an injury of the cervical spine. J Bone Joint Surg 1989;71-A:15–22.
24 Swain A, Grundy D, Russell J: ABC of spinal cord injury: Evacuation and initial management at hospital. Br Med J 1985;291: 1623–1625.
25 Sneed RC, Stover SL: Undiagnosed spinal cord injuries in brain-injured children. Am J Dis Child 1988;142:965–967.
26 Kendall KP, McCreary EK: Muscles: Testing and Function. Baltimore, Williams & Wilkins, 1983.
27 American Spinal Injury Association: Standards for Neurological Classification of Spinal Injury Patients. Chicago, ASIA, 1989.
28 Stauffer ES: Diagnosis and prognosis of acute cervical spinal cord injury. Clin Orthop 1975;112:9–15.
29 Janssen L, Hansebout RR: Pathogenesis of spinal cord injury and newer treatments: A review. Spine 1989;14:23–32.
30 Feldman F: CT and spinal column injury. Orthop Rev 1983;12: 49–55.
31 Cooperman LH: Succinylcholine-induced hyperkalemia in neuromuscular disease. JAMA 1970;213:1867–1871.
32 Waters RL, Adkins RH, Nelson R, et al: Cervical spinal cord trauma: Evaluation and non-operative treatment with halo-vest immobilization. Contemp Orthop 1987;14:35–45.
33 Bohlman HH: Current concepts review: Treatment of fractures and dislocations of the thoracic and lumbar spine. J Bone Joint Surg 1987;67-A:165–169.
34 Young JS, Burns PE, Bowen AM, et al: Spinal Cord Injury Statistics: Experience of the Regional Spinal Cord Injury Systems. Phoenix, Good Samaritan Medical Center, 1982.
35 Glenn WWL, Hogan JF, Loke JSO, et al: Ventilatory support by pacing of the conditioned diaphragm in quadriplegia. N Engl J Med 1984;310:1150–1155.
36 Miller HJ, Thomas E, Wilmot CB: Pneumobelt use among high quadriplegic population. Arch Phys Med Rehabil 1988;69:369–372.
37 Levine SP, Koester DJ, Kett RL: Independently activated talking tracheostomy systems for quadriplegic patients. Arch Phys Med Rehabil 1987;68:571–573.
38 Carter RE, Donovan WH, Halstead L, et al: Comparative study of electrophrenic nerve stimulation and mechanical ventilatory support in traumatic spinal cord injury. Paraplegia 1987;25:86–91.
39 Goldberg AI, Monahan CA: Home health care for children assisted by mechanical ventilation: The physician's perspective. J Pediatr 1989;114:378–383.
40 Cahill JL, Okamoto GA, Higgins T, et al: Experiences with phrenic nerve pacing in children. J Pediatr Surg 1983;18:851–854.
41 Light JK, Scott FB: The artificial urinary sphincter in children. Br J Urol 1984;56:54–57.
42 Kimura DK, Mayo M, Shurtleff D: Urinary tract management; in Shurtleff DB (ed): Myelodysplasias and Extrophies: Significance, Prevention, and Treatment. New York, Grune & Stratton, 1986.
43 Maynard FM, Diokno AC: Urinary infection and complications during clean intermittent catheterization following spinal cord injury. J Urol 1984;132:943–946.
44 Koff SA: Estimating bladder capacity in children. Urology 1983; 21:248.
45 Fisher SV, Gullickson G: Energy cost of ambulation in health and disability: A literature review. Arch Phys Med Rehabil 1978;59:124–133.
46 Brittell CW, Johnson DR, Ciciora J: Unistick vehicle controller: A unique approach to driving for severely handicapped individuals. Arch Phys Med Rehabil 1984;65:664.
47 Pollack SF, Axen K, Spielholz N, et al: Aerobic training effects of electrically induced lower extremity exercises in spinal cord injured people. Arch Phys Med Rehabil 1989;70:214–219.
48 Turk R, Obreza P: Functional electrical stimulation as an orthotic means for the rehabilitation of paraplegic patients. Paraplegia 1985;23:344–348.
49 Griffith ER, Tomko MA, Timms RJ: Sexual function in spinal cord injured patients. A review. Arch Phys Med Rehabil 1973; 54:539–543.
50 Berczeller PH, Bezkor MF: Medical Complications of Quadriplegia. Chicago, Year Book Medical Publishers, 1986.
51 Mahoney FP: Pulmonary function in quadriplegia: Effects of a corset. Arch Phys Med Rehabil 1979;60:261–265.
52 Gilgoff IS, Barras DM, Jones MS, et al: Neck breathing: A form of voluntary respiration for the spine injured ventilator-dependent child. Pediatrics 1988;82:741–745.
53 Gross D, Ladd HW, Riley EJ: The effect of training on strength and endurance of the diaphragm in quadriplegia. Am J Med 1980;68:27–35.
54 Sayegh A: Intermittent pneumatic compression: Past, present and future. Clin Rehabil 1987;1:59–64.
55 Erickson RP: Autonomic hyperreflexia: Pathophysiology and medical management. Arch Phys Med Rehabil 1980;61:431–440.
56 Katz RT, Rymer WZ: Spastic hypertonia: Mechanisms and measurement. Arch Phys Med Rehabil 1989;70:144–155.
57 LaHaye PA, Batzdorf U: Posttraumatic syringomyelia. West J Med 1988;148:657–663.
58 Mohler JL, Cowen DL, Flanigan RC: Suppression and treatment of urinary tract infection in patients with an intermittently catheterized neurogenic bladder. J Urol 1987;138:336–340.
59 Stover SL, Lloyd LK, Waites KB, et al: Urinary tract infection in spinal cord injury. Arch Phys Med Rehabil 1989;70:47–54.
60 Lebowitz RL: Pediatric uroradiology. Pediatr Clin North Am 1985;32:1353–1362.
61 VanZuiden L, Anquist KA, Schachar N, et al: Immobilization hypercalcemia. Can J Surg 1982;25:646–649.
62 Merli GJ, McElwain GE, Adler AG, et al: Immobilization hypercalcemia in acute spinal cord injury treated with etidronate. Arch Intern Med 1984;144:1286–1288.
63 Grundy D, Russell J: ABC of spinal cord injury: Medical management in the spinal injuries unit. Br Med J 1986;292:183–187.
64 Weitzman M: School and peer relations. Pediatr Clin North Am 1984;31:59–69.

Received: June 1, 1989

Teresa L. Massagli, MD
Department of Rehabilitation Medicine
University of Washington School of Medicine
Children's Hospital and Medical Center
P.O. Box C5371, Seattle, WA 98105 (USA)

Pediatrician 1990;17:255–261

0300–1245/90/0174–0255$2.75/0

Psychosocial Consequences of Head Injury in Children and Adolescents: Implications for Rehabilitation

M.G. Livingston[a], *R.J.R. McCabe*[b]

[a] Department of Psychological Medicine, University of Glasgow; [b] Adolescent Unit, Gartnavel Royal Hospital, Glasgow, Scotland

Key Words. Head injury · Children · Adolescents · Psychosocial · Rehabilitation

Abstract. Studies measuring psychosocial outcome in children and adolescents have shown that head injury leads to cognitive impairment which is directly related to the severity of injury in those with very severe head injury. Psychiatric disorders are also related to the severity of injury but here the relationship suggests that mediating factors are involved. No specific pattern of post-traumatic psychological/psychiatric dysfunction emerges from the studies, but it is clear that, as with adults, psychosocial recovery lags behind physical. Head injury affects the functioning of the young person in the family, at school, and within the wider community, often resulting in a secondary handicap of low self-esteem. The multitude of deficits which are a consequence of severe head injury present a challenge for rehabilitation specialists. A multi-disciplinary, multi-specialist, and multi-agency response is required. As a result, families are often presented with a bewildering array of treatments and programmes at different agencies. A case manager can be helpful in ensuring the appropriate use of available resources and can be the one professional in charge of a coordinating case record.

Introduction

Accidents are the leading cause of morbidity and mortality during childhood [1]. Although statistics are hard to obtain because it is often difficult to separate head injury referrals from other trauma victims, 200,000 children receive hospital treatment for head injury each year in the US [2]. Of these, 4,000 die and 15,000 require prolonged hospital treatment and rehabilitation.

The highest incidence of head injury is in the 15–24 age group. Most falls occur in those aged under 15 [3]. There is a vast cost to health services as a result. Rune [4] assessed that 15% of the population in a medium-size Swedish town who are aged between 7 and 16 years would experience a head injury. A quarter of those who receive hospital treatment for head injury in England and Wales are children of school age [5] and the numbers have been rising steadily since the fifties [6].

Head trauma in children is, therefore, a major health issue. A wide variety of physical, social and psychological consequences present a challenge to rehabilitation specialists.

The causes of head injury in children are many and have been listed according to age-based vulnerability [7]. Infants often are injured as a result of accidental dropping or as a consequence of deliberate abuse. Young children of toddler or pre-school age suffer falls, or again are victims of abuse. Older children sustain injuries as passengers in cars or as pedestrians. By the time schooling has commenced, sports and recreational activities feature as causes, and in the adolescent drugs, alcohol, driving accidents, and assaults become prominent.

Children and adolescents who injure themselves severely often come from families in which there is considerable psychosocial disadvantage. The pattern is similar to adults with severe head injury, where victims are

Table 1. Glasgow assessment schedule

Assess		Scoring
Personality change		
Emotional lability		NMS – 0, 1, 2
Irritability		NMS – 0, 1, 2
Aggressiveness		NMS – 0, 1, 2
Any other behavioural change (ask patient, obtain corroboration from relatives)		NMS – 0, 1, 2
Subjective complaints		
Sleep disturbance		NMS – 0, 1, 2
Incontinence		NMS – 0, 1, 2
Family stress		NMS – 0, 1, 2
Financial problems		NMS – 0, 1, 2
Sexual problems		NMS – 0, 1, 2
Alcohol, excess drinking or poor tolerance		NMS – 0, 1, 2
Reduced leisure and sporting activities		NMS – 0, 1, 2
Headache		NMS – 0, 1, 2
Dizziness, loss of balance		NMS – 0, 1, 2
Parasthesia		NMS – 0, 1, 2
Reduced sense of smell		NMS – 0, 1, 2
Reduced hearing		NMS – 0, 1, 2
Reduced vision (ask patient, obtain corroboration from relatives)		NMS – 0, 1, 2
Occupational functioning		
At work	same job	0
	similar job	0
	less skilled job	1
Not at work	employable	2
	unemployable	3

Assess		Scoring
Cognitive functioning		
Immediate recall		
name, address, telephone number		NMS – 0, 1, 2
Two-minute recall		
name, address, telephone number		NMS – 0, 1, 2
Attention and concentration – serial 7's subtracted from 100 or serial 3's subtracted from 20		NMS – 0, 1, 2
Orientation – time, place and person		NMS – 0, 1, 2
Current intelligence status		
simple, arithmetic and general knowledge questions		
normal, borderline-defective, defective		NMS – 0, 1, 2
Physical examination		
Dysphasia		NMS – 0, 1, 2
Dysarthria		NMS – 0, 1, 2
Abnormal muscle tone – right leg		NMS – 0, 1, 2
Abnormal muscle tone – left leg		NMS – 0, 1, 2
Abnormal muscle tone – upper limbs		NMS – 0, 1, 2
Walking		NMS – 0, 1, 2
Cranial nerve deficits		NMS – 0, 1, 2
Seizures		NMS – 0, 1, 2
Activities of daily living		
Cooking	OO, WH, UTM	0, 1, 2
Other domestic tasks	OO, WH, UTM	0, 1, 2
Shopping	OO, WH, UTM	0, 1, 2
Travelling	OO, WH, UTM	0, 1, 2
Personal hygiene	OO, WH, UTM	0, 1, 2
Feeding	OO, WH, UTM	0, 1, 2
Dressing	OO, WH, UTM	0, 1, 2
Mobility	OO, WH, UTM	0, 1, 2

NMS = Normal, moderate severity, severe; OO = On own; WH = with help; UTM = unable to manage.

more commonly males of lower socio-economic status with a history of risk taking and alcoholic over-indulgence [8].

Assessment and Methodology

Special problems occur in the assessment of children with head injury. In small children, the level of language attainment determines the type of testing which can be carried out. The assessment of post-traumatic amnesia (PTA) [9], vital as a severity measure in adults, is often highly inaccurate in children. The clinician, therefore, more frequently depends on the accounts of parents and therapeutic staff. Furthermore, the child is undergoing dynamic development in a cognitive sense; outcome studies require age-matched controls. Is development impeded by the injury? Is this normal progress? These questions are difficult to answer, because a child's cognitive attainment may normally proceed in a step-wise fashion, rather than by smooth acquisition.

The measurement of outcome in head injury is essential for documenting progress. This process not only sets out what has been achieved, but can act as positive reinforcement to the therapeutic endeavours of staff, patient and family. The assessment of outcome has, in the past, all too frequently focused exclusively on physical restitution or on global measures of disability [10]. This approach fails to meet the needs of the head injury victim for a comprehensive rehabilitation approach which addresses psychosocial factors as well as the physical consequences of the injury.

Table 2. Severe and mild head injury compared to orthopaedic injuries not involving the head [adapted from ref. 16]

Clinical characteristics		Severe head injury	Mild head injury	Orthopaedic patients without head injury
Patients, n		31	29	28
PTA		> 7 days	> 1 h < 6 days	none
Assessment intervals		soon after injury 4 months 12 months 2¼ years	soon after injury 4 months 12 months 2¼ years	soon after injury 4 months 12 months 2¼ years
Measures	Children	psychometric testing – WISC – Neale reading analysis – specific cognitive test neurological examination (only at final assessment)	psychometric testing – WISC – Neale reading analysis – specific cognitive test	psychometric testing – WISC – Neale reading analysis – specific cognitive test
	Parents	standardised interview	standardised interview	standardised interview
	Parents and teachers	behavioural questionnaire	behavioural questionnaire	behavioural questionnaire

WISC = Wechsler intelligence scale for children.

These factors have led to the development of rating instruments for assessing all aspects of outcome; e.g. the Glasgow assessment schedule [11]. Essentially, this instrument enables scores to be derived for physical, psychological, and social outcome, together with a global outcome score. These ratings can be used to record outcome cross-sectionally, and over time enable a reliable measure of outcome to be ascertained in rehabilitation programmes. This instrument is illustrated in table 1. It was devised with adult head-injured subjects in mind and its psychometric properties to date have been assessed with this group. With some adaptation, the scale might be useful in children and adolescents. Clearly, the activities of daily living and cognitive assessments would require particular orientation towards the needs of such a population and the occupational functioning scale could be related to schooling or education.

Physical Outcome

Some reports suggest that head injury mortality is low in children [12]. Patient selection often plays a part in such figures, excluding patients who failed to survive before arriving at the neurosurgical centre. In the series of Berger et al. [13], a consecutive sample of 37 young people under the age of 17 who had suffered a head injury was examined; 33% had died, 2% remained in a 'vegetative state' and 14% had a poor outcome. There was no significant relationship between age and outcome, but the sample of very young children was small and these children may be at special risk in terms of outcome. The study suggests a more favourable outcome for children after head injury.

In children and adolescents, as with adults [14], the major physical consequences of head injury are orthopaedic deficits, and neurological problems including sensory deficits such as impaired hearing, smell and vision. Together with epilepsy, they contribute to cognitive impairment as well as inducing negative self-image [15]. This is especially important for older children and adolescents where the peer group may reject, stigmatise, or taunt a young person with obvious physical handicaps. Thus, physical status may be crucial for determining the psychosocial outcome and for understanding the coping strategy of the head-injured child/adolescent.

Rutter et al. [16] compared controls (orthopaedic injuries not involving the head) with mildly and severely injured head trauma children. The characteristics of the population and the measurements carried out are summarised in table 2.

At the 4-month assessment, 6 controls had motor deficits. The mildly injured children had few physical problems, but 13 severely injured had motor, visual, auditory and speech deficits. At the 27-month assessment, there were no further problems in this with a minor injury, but the more severely injured patients had continuing handicaps. These included hemiplegia, dysarthria, facial weakness, and several had speech, hearing and visual problems. Fourteen of the 29 severely injured patients had a neurological finding at the 27-month assessment: 2 cranial nerve lesions, 4 children with incoordination of posture and gait, 6 with unilateral signs of hemiparesis and 2 with signs of bilateral cerebral involvement. No child had persistent post-traumatic seizures, although 6 had fits between the end of the acute admission phase and the 4-month review.

Cognitive Impairment

A number of studies have shown scholastic and intellectual impairment following severe head injury in children [17–20]. The literature repeatedly reports that the more severe injuries, as assessed by coma measures (e.g. GCS [21] or PTA), are more likely to result in such impairment.

Levin and Eisenberg [18] demonstrated significant impairment detectable at 12-month follow-up in 45 children and adolescents after severe head injury (coma $>$ 24 h). Black et al. [22, 23] described a 5-year prospective study of mild and severe head injury children. The children showed gradual cognitive improvement, but since there were no controls, a practice effect may have contributed to the results. Klonoff et al. [24] in a controlled study showed that 5 years after injury less than 25% showed neuropsychological impairment on their test battery. Those who were impaired were mainly severe head injuries; but 50% of the subjects were lost to follow-up.

In adults, verbal skills which are 'overlearned' tend to be less affected than visuo-spatial skills [10]. In children, verbal deficits may be more affected in the long term [23]. Age has little impact on recovery from head injury in children [18, 24] except that the very young (under 4 years) do very badly.

Rutter et al. [16] argued the need for studies with matched control groups and a prospective design to assess whether a causal link between head injury and cognitive impairment exists. Such a design was employed in their series which involved follow-up of head-injured children for 2¼ years [25]. The sample consisted of 31 children with PTA greater than 7 days, 28 individually matched orthopaedic controls, and 29 mild head injuries with PTA between 1 h and 7 days. Psychological tests were carried out at 4, 12 and 27 months using the Wechsler intelligence scale for children, the Neale analysis of reading ability, together with other more specific cognitive tests.

There was some cognitive impairment in children with mild injury, which failed to recover, and thus was presumed to be non-organically based. In the severely injured children, cognitive impairment was particularly evident where PTA was greater than 2 weeks. The impairment was greater for the most severely injured and recovered, implying a causal relationship between injury and cognitive deficit. Timed measures of visuo-spatial and visuo-motor skills were more likely to be affected than verbal skills, but no specific pattern of cognitive impairments emerged. Subsequently Winogron et al. [26] showed that the most severely injured children (GCS ≤ 7) were handicapped on timed performance, visuo-motor tests, and on a verbal fluency measure compared with mild and moderately injured children. The pattern of deficits was more distinctive in those with the more severe injuries.

Although the evidence for a specific cognitive syndrome following head injury is equivocal, it is clear that recovery is rapid in the first few months for the 'organically' based impairments, and continues for at least 12–24 months. Age, sex and social class of the child were not linked to recovery [25]. Head injury rarely retarded scholastic achievement unless PTA exceeded 3 weeks.

Language impairment may occur in children after severe head injury with naming, expressive and written language skills more likely to be impaired than receptive functions [27]. Children's written language skills were more adversely affected than those of adolescents. Clearly such impairments affect psychological testing which depends on language skills for performance.

Psychiatric Outcome

This field has been reviewed by Lishman [28, 29] for adults after head injury where the main sequels are personality change and post-traumatic neurotic dysfunction. Psychotic disturbance is more rare, and when it occurs paranoid illnesses are the commonest. In children, disturbed behaviour tends to be the most frequent sequel.

The Rutter Isle of Wight study has become a classic of the child psychiatry literature [30]. This study reviewed children within an entire community, and showed that children of normal intelligence with organic brain damage were twice as likely to show behavioural disturbance. Since many such children have visible handicaps, as a result of their disorder (e.g. hemiplegia), it was necessary to replicate this finding using a control group suffering from similar handicaps [31] which did not involve lesions of the central nervous system. The findings were confirmed, leading to an expectation of similar results (behavioural disturbances) in those children who have sustained traumatic cerebral insult.

In head injury studies, cause and effect often are hard to separate: deviant and disadvantaged children more frequently injure their heads which leads to behavioural problems. Brown et al. [32] controlled for such adversity by matching patients with head injury with a group of 28 accident/orthopaedic children without head injury, using a prospective design. Information was collected from the parents using a semi-structured interview [33, 34] and from schools and teachers (Rutter B_2 scale) [35]. Although a clear link between length of PTA and severity of psychiatric disturbance was not shown, children with PTAs of longer than 2–3 weeks were at particular risk. This suggests that psychiatric disorder following head injury, unlike cognitive impairment, may be mediated by other factors, possibly in a manner which has been postulated for depression [36].

Psychiatric difficulties after head injury were linked to pre-accident behaviour, intelligence, and psychosocial circumstances. Age (bearing in mind that the sample did not contain very young poor-prognosis children) was not associated with psychiatric dysfunction, nor were the sex of the child or the nature and degree of physical injury. Disinhibition, increased emotionality, and mixtures of these two syndromes were common. The only example of psychosis occurred in a 15-year-old.

Assessment for Rehabilitation

Children and adolescents with severe head injury often sustain multiple handicaps. Such handicaps necessitate a multi-disciplinary, multi-agency approach to assessment and management. Chorazy [37] has emphasised the need to see the child as a 'whole person' and thus to avoid a piecemeal approach to rehabilitation. In some agencies, a case manager coordinates the rehabilitation effort for the child and family.

For children and adolescents there are three social settings of importance: the family, the place of education, and the wider community, including the relevant peer group. A coordinated rehabilitation programme will involve not only the appropriate medical and paramedical disciplines within the hospital setting, but also educational psychology and social work.

In work with brain injured adults, standardised assessment techniques are frequently employed. There is a need to develop instruments for use with children and adolescents which not only measure deficits such as cognitive impairment, but which also assess the need for rehabilitation and measure outcome.

Rehabilitation Techniques

General principles of rehabilitation include: (1) acceptance of attenuated daily living skills; (2) need to develop compensatory coping strategies; (3) need to reward effort as well as achievement; (4) need to set realistic targets; (5) reinforcement of the residual strengths of the child/adolescent, and (6) need to tackle negative self-defeating attitudes in the child and family [15].

Many rehabilitation schemes exist, but few have been evaluated [38, 39]. Programmes are often put together on an ad hoc basis, dependent on the available skills and enthusiasm. Two main therapeutic techniques are employed to deal with the psychosocial consequences of head injury in children: cognitive/behavioural and psychodynamic.

Cognitive/behavioural approaches involve learning adaptive patterns of behaviour and attempting to extinguish maladaptive 'coping' strategies. Behaviours which may need to be tackled include disinhibition, emotionality, and hyperactivity [32]. In addition, there are a variety of cognitive programmes, often computer assisted, for retraining impaired memory, concentration and learning skills.

In psychodynamic work, the aim is to promote insight and possibly the acceptance of new limitations. Coping with grieving over the loss of function is a major theme, often addressing the denial of difficulties and problems by the young person and the family. This approach is of particular relevance to the adolescent where there is a struggle to develop a post-injury identity.

In both of these approaches, directive- and insight-based, therapists have to counter negative self-concepts and, at the same time, be aware of the capacity of the brain-injured person to learn and to adapt. Group work as well as individual counseling is necessary. The brain-injured child/adolescent has to re-learn how to integrate within a relevant peer group. The therapist's task is to encourage the development of pro-social functioning, promoting an optimum social identity.

Families

The burden on families of the adult brain injured has been well documented and a number of studies have provided objective measures of the impact on the relatives [40]. In working with such families facing handicap in their midst, Black [41] has set two objectives: maintaining a cohesive supportive family and encouraging the young person to optimal achievement.

Families are sometimes misled by the early encouraging improvements in physical health, only to have their hopes dashed by the continuing toll of psychosocial difficulties. The family's process of adaptation to the reality of brain injury has been compared with grief and mourning [41], but such families must learn to cope with an ever-changing situation unlike the finality of death, a situation termed 'mobile mourning' [42].

Families may cope by being over-restrictive, over-protective and by seeking too readily to appease the child. The needs of the parents and of other siblings are all too easily over-looked. A family therapy approach, which is eclectic, flexible and imaginative, can help work with these problems and may provide an opportunity for the family to grow together through the common experience of tragedy.

References

1 United States National Center for Health Statistics: Facts of life and death. DHEW Publ. PHS 79-1222, United States Public Health Service, Hyattsville (1978).

2 Mahoney, W.J.; D'Souza, B.J.; Haller, J.A.; et al.: Long-term outcome of children with severe head trauma and prolonged coma. Pediatrics *71:* 756–762 (1983).

3 Kalsbeek, W.D.; McLaurin, R.L.; Harris, B.S.H.; et al.: The national head and spinal cord injury survey. J. Neurosurg. *53:* 19–31 (1980).

4 Rune, V.: Acute head injuries in children. Acta psychiat. scand., suppl. 209, pp. 3–12 (1970).

5 Field, J.H.: Epidemiology of head injury in England and Wales. (HMSO, London 1976).

6 Craft, A.W.; Shaw, D.A.; Cartiledge, N.E.: Head injuries in children. Br. med. J. *iii:* 200–203 (1972).

7 Rivara, F.P.: Childhood injuries. III. Epidemiology of non-motor vehicle trauma. Dev. Med. Child Neur. *26:* 81–87 (1984).

8 Galbraith, S.; Murray, W.R.; Patel, A.R.; et al.: The relationship between alcohol and head injury and its effect on the conscious level. Br. J. Surg. *63:* 127–130 (1976).

9 Russell, W.R.; Nathan, P.W.: Traumatic amnesia. Brain *69:* 280–300 (1946).

10 Bond, M.R.: Assessment of psychosocial outcome of severe head injury. Acta neurochir. *31:* 51–70 (1976).

11 Livingston, M.G.; Livingston, H.M.: The Glasgow assessment schedule. Int. Rehabil. Med. *7:* 145–149 (1985).

12 Bruce, D.A.; Schut, L.; Bruno, L.; et al.: Outcome following severe head injuries in children. J. Neurosurg. *48:* 679–688 (1978).

13 Berger, M.S.; Pitts, L.H.; Lovely, M.; et al.: Outcome from severe head injury in children and adolescents. J. Neurosurg. *62:* 194–199 (1985).

14 Jennett, B.; Snoek, J.; Bond, M.R.; et al.: Disability after severe head injury: observations on the use of the Glasgow outcome scale. J. Neurol. Neurosurg. Psychiat. *44:* 285–293 (1981).

15 McCabe, R.J.R.; Green, D.: Rehabilitating severely head-injured adolescents: three case reports. J. Child. Psychol. Psychiat. *28:* 111–126 (1987).

16 Rutter, M.; Chadwick, O.; Shaffer, D.; et al.: A prospective study of children with head injuries: I. Design and methods. Psychol. Med. *10:* 633–645 (1980).

17 Brink, J.D.; Garrett, A.L.; Hale, W.R.; et al.: Recovery of motor and intellectual function in children sustaining severe head injuries. Devl Med. Child Neur. *12:* 545–572 (1970).

18 Levin, H.S.; Eisenberg, H.M.: Neuropsychological outcome of closed head injury in children and adolescents. Child's Brain *5:* 281–292 (1979).

19 Richardson, F.: Some effects of severe head injury: a follow-up study of children and adolescents after protracted coma. Devl Med. Child Neur. *5:* 471–482 (1963).

20 Heiskanen, D.; Kaste, M.: Late prognosis of severe brain injury in children. Devl Med. Child Neur. *16:* 11–14 (1974).

21 Teasdale, G.; Jennett, B.: Assessment of coma and impaired consciousness. Lancet *ii:* 81–84 (1974).

22 Black, P.; Jeffries, J.; Blumer, D.; et al.: The post-traumatic syndrome in children: characteristics and incidence; in Walker, Caveness, The late effects of head injury, pp. 142–149 (Thomas, Springfield 1969).

23 Black, P.; Blumer, D.; Wellner, A.M.; et al.: The head injured child: time course of recovery with implications for rehabilitation; in Head injuries, pp. 131–137. Proc. Int. Symp. Edinburgh, Madrid 1970. (Williams and Wilkins, Baltimore 1970).

24 Klonoff, H.; Low, M.D.; Clark, C.: Head injuries in children: a prospective 5-year follow-up. J. Neurol. Neurosurg. Psychiat. *40:* 1211–1219 (1977).

25 Chadwick, O.; Rutter, M.; Shaffer, D.; et al.: A prospective study of children with head injuries. IV. Cognitive deficits. J. consult. clin. Neuropsychol. *3:* 101–120 (1981).

26 Winogron, H.W.; Knights, R.M.; Brandon, H.N.: Neuropsychological deficits following head injury in children. J. clin. Neuropsychol. *6:* 269–286 (1984).

27 Ewing-Cobbs, L.; Levin, S.; Eisenberg, H.M.; et al.: Language functions following closed head injury in children and adolescents. J. clin. exp. Neuropsychol. *9:* 575–592 (1987).

28 Lishman, W.A.: Brain damage in relation to psychiatric disability after head injury. Br. J. Psychiat. *114:* 373–410 (1968).
29 Lishman, W.A.: Psychiatric sequelae of head injury: a review. Psychol. Med. *3:* 304–318 (1973).
30 Rutter, M.; Graham, P.; Yule, W.: A neuropsychiatric study in childhood. Clinics in developmental medicine No. 35–36 (Heineman Medical Books, London 1970).
31 Seidal, U.; Chadwick, O.; Rutter, M.: Psychiatric disorders in crippled children. A comparative study of children with and without brain damage. Devl Med. Child Neur. *17:* 563–573 (1975).
32 Brown, G.; Chadwick, O.; Shaffer, D.; et al.: A prospective study of children with severe head injuries. III. Psychiatric sequelae. Psychol. Med. *11:* 63–78 (1981).
33 Brown, G.W.; Rutter, M.: The assessment of family activities and relationships: a methodological study. Hum. Relat. *19:* 241–263 (1966).
34 Rutter, M.; Brown, G.W.: The reliability and validity of measures of family life and relationships in families containing a psychiatric patient. Soc. Psychiatr. *1:* 38–53 (1966).
35 Rutter, M.: A children's behaviour questionnaire for completion by teachers: preliminary findings. J. Child Psychol. Psychiat. *8:* 1–11 (1967).
36 Brown, G.W.; Harris, T.O.; Copeland, J.R.: Depression and loss. Br. J. Psychiat. *129:* 125–137 (1976).
37 Chorazy, A.J.L.: Introduction; in Ylvisaker, Head injury rehabilitation (College Hill Press, San Diego 1985).
38 Pond, D.A.: Residential psychiatric treatment of children with epilepsy and brain damage; in Barker, The residential psychiatric treatment of children, pp. 235–257 (Crosby Lockwood Staples, London 1974).
39 Ylvisaker, M.: Head injury rehabilitation: children and adults (College Hill Press, San Diego 1985).
40 Livingston, M.G.; Brooks, D.N.: The burden on families of the brain injured: a review. J. Head Trauma Rehabil. *3:* 6–15 (1988).
41 Black, D.: Handicap and family therapy; in Bentovin, Gorell-Barnes, Cooklin, Family therapy, vol. II, Complementary framework of theory and practice, pp. 417–439 (Academic Press, London 1982).
42 Rosenthal, M.; Muir, C.A.: Methods of family education; in Rosenthal, Griffith, Miller, Rehabilitation of the head-injured adult, pp. 407–419 (Davis, Philadelphia 1983).

Received: September 14, 1989

M.G. Livingston, MD
Department of Psychological Medicine
University of Glasgow
6 Whittingehame Gardens
Great Western Road
Glasgow, G12 0AA (Scotland)

Pediatrician 1990;17:262–266

0300–1245/90/0174–0262$2.75/0

Rehabilitation of the Injured Athlete

Terry L. Thompson, Elliott B. Hershman, James A. Nicholas

Nicholas Institute of Sports Medicine and Athletic Trauma, Lenox Hill Hospital, New York, N.Y., USA

Key Words. Athletic injuries · Sports medicine · Rehabilitation

Abstract. An increase in the rate of injuries has accompanied the boom in sports participation among children and adolescents. Accurate diagnosis, prompt treatment, and comprehensive rehabilitation are keys to the safe return of the young athlete to sports. Reacquisition of flexibility, strength, and endurance forms the basis of reconditioning. A graded reacclimatization to the demands of the sport allows the athlete to attain the preinjury level of skill. Psychological ramifications of injury such as fear, anger, and depression are to be expected and must be dealt with appropriately.

Introduction

Youth participation in sports on both a recreational and competitive level has increased dramatically over the past 30 years. This has done much to enhance the general health and well-being of children. Unfortunately, along with this rise in participation has come an increase in sports-related injuries. Although children have an enormous capacity for healing, appropriate rehabilitation of sports-related injuries must be undertaken with the same vigor as with their adult counterparts. Factors unique to the immature athlete must be considered during the course of rehabilitation.

Team Approach

A team approach is essential to comprehensive sports injury rehabilitation. No one health professional can effectively provide all services needed by the recovering athlete. The physician, physical therapist, trainer, and coach should work closely together in the rehabilitation process. The rehabilitation plan must be prescribed and coordinated by the physician. The progress of the athlete should be frequently monitored, as alterations in the program may be necessary.

Linkage

In the rehabilitation of any athletic injury the concept of linkage must be kept in mind [1]. A significant injury to any component of the musculoskeletal system will invariably have an impact on structures proximal and distal to the site of injury. Secondary effects also occur in the cardiovascular, neurological, and other organ systems. If attention is focused solely on the site of injury, complete recovery is compromised. Further, the demands of the chosen sport may not be met because of residual deficits in the musculoskeletal system away from the site of injury. With ‘total body linkage’ as a basis, a rational and comprehensive approach to rehabilitation may be taken.

Components of Athletic Rehabilitation

Rehabilitation ideally begins immediately after injury and ends when the athlete returns to full activity without limitations imposed by the injury [2]. Treatment of the injury and some degree of healing must precede reconditioning. Therefore, treatment and healing become integral parts of the rehabilitation process. Following injury, anatomical restoration of damaged structures becomes the primary goal. This may be accomplished by nonoperative or operative methods. Rest and immobilization are often required to facilitate the healing process. Muscle atrophy is a consequence of limb immobilization. Maintaining muscle in the lengthened position, isometric muscle contractions, and electrical muscle stimulation are useful ways to decrease muscle atrophy during immobilization [3]. During the early healing phase the athlete should be encouraged to perform strengthening and endurance exercises using body parts not affected by the injury. These measures will shorten recovery.

Pain is a natural sequela of injury and is usually present to some degree during the early phases of healing. Pain activates neural mechanisms which initiate muscle function, making it difficult for the injured athlete to perform exercises that are essential for a speedy recovery. Judicious use of analgesics and therapeutic modalities such as cryotherapy and heat help provide necessary pain relief.

The essential components of any athletic reconditioning program will include measures to restore flexibility, strength, and cardiovascular endurance. Kegerreis [4] has used 'functional progressions' in the augmentation of traditional athletic rehabilitation to achieve complete restoration of athletic abilities. Functional progression is defined as an ordered sequence of activities enabling the acquisition or reacquisition of skills required for the safe, effective performance of the chosen sport. If this important component of rehabilitation is omitted, the athlete may be physically fit but may lack the confidence to return to full sports participation.

Flexibility

Flexibility is the ability to move unresisted through a full range of motion and is as important to an athlete as strength, cardiovascular conditioning or timing [3]. Joints and muscles may lose flexibility in response to injury and immobilization. Flexibility has primary importance in rehabilitation in that the fullest muscle-tendon length gives a more efficient contraction [5]. Efforts should be made to begin early motion in injured joints as soon after injury or surgery as is safely possible [6].

When immobilization is discontinued or when restrictions on range of motion are removed, stretching exercises may be initiated. Stretching exercises use forced motion applied actively by the individual contracting the antagonist muscle group or passively by an external force stretching the muscle [7]. There are three types of stretching: static, ballistic and proprioceptive neuromuscular facilitation.

Static stretching is the most commonly used method. It is performed by holding the muscle in a lengthened position for a period of time, followed by relaxation. Several repetitions are done, with the idea of increasing excursion with each successive effort.

In ballistic stretching the position of stretch is assumed and a bouncing motion is utilized. This method is often more painful and even may result in muscle tears if the tolerance of the muscle being stretched is exceeded [8].

Proprioceptive neuromuscular facilitation techniques require a partner. Increased flexibility is gained by first fatiguing the muscle by requiring it to contract isometrically for a period of time against a fixed resistance (fig. 1a). The muscle is then relaxed, and the antagonist contracts along with assisted movement from the partner [8] (fig. 1b). This technique is not only useful in rehabilitation but may also be used in injury prevention and warm-up [9].

Strength

Delorme [10] popularized the use of heavy resistance exercises to restore muscle power after injury during the 1940s. Since that time, numerous strength programs and types of exercise equipment have been developed that have revolutionized sports injury rehabilitation. Although strength training in children remains a controversial issue, there is a growing body of evidence that supports its safety and efficacy [11]. There are three types of strength training modalities: isometric, isotonic, and isokinetic. A working understanding of each will allow for its proper use in prescribing a rehabilitation program.

Isometric exercise involves contraction of a muscle against a fixed resistance such that no joint motion occurs. The muscle unit may be loaded maximally; however, since the muscle is only loaded at one point in the range of motion of the joint, there is little effect on motor performance [12]. Therefore, isometrics have limited use as a singular strength modality in athletic rehabilitation. Isometric exercise may be useful in the early stages of rehabilitation when the limb is immobilized or in the treatment of knee injuries when the lack of patellar loading is desirable [13].

Isotonic exercise is done through a full range of motion with a fixed resistance. An isotonic muscle contraction may be concentric, in which the muscle shortens

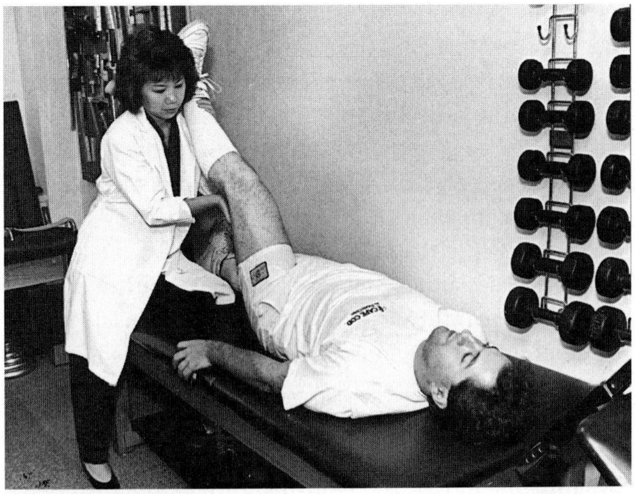

1a

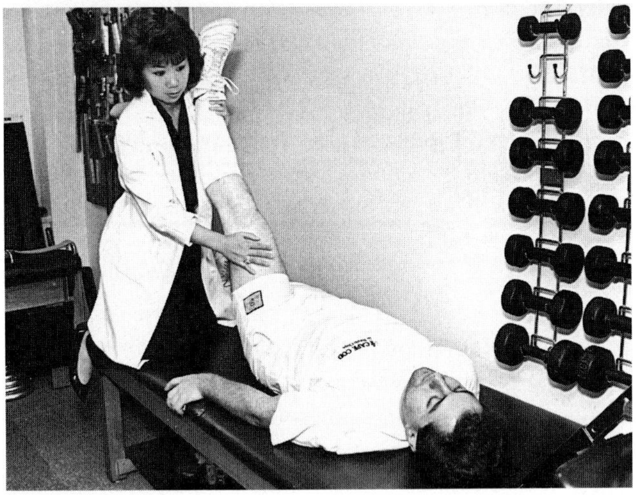

1b

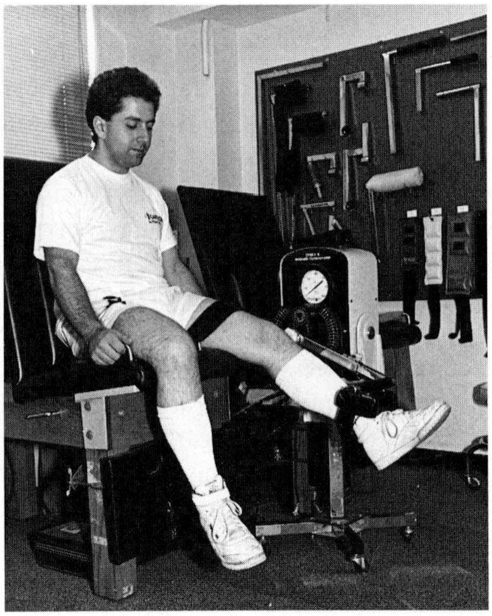

2

Fig. 1. Technique of proprioceptive neuromuscular facilitation stretching. **a** Contract phase – athlete contracts hamstring with physical therapist applying resistance. **b** Relax/stretch phase – therapist stretches hamstring passively.

Fig. 2. Isokinetic strength work is performed on Cybex dynamometer. Both hamstring and quadriceps strengthening is performed by sequential contraction of knee flexors and extensors.

against resistance, or eccentric, in which the muscle lengthens. Equipment for isotonic exercises is simple and readily available. The most common example is free weights. A disadvantage of free weights is that the force on the muscle is not constant through a full range of motion. The muscle is loaded maximally only at its weakest point, and the rest of the system is operating at less than capacity [12]. A variation of isotonic exercise called variable resistance (Nautilus®, Eagle®) attempts to provide maximum resistance throughout the range of motion by employing cams and pulleys.

Isokinetic exercise is performed at a fixed speed with resistance that is accommodating throughout a range of motion (fig. 2). Isokinetics have proven to be a useful therapeutic tool because of three unique features [14]. (1) Maximal dynamic loading of a muscle may be achieved throughout a range of motion. (2) Resistance is accommodating; therefore, a patient may use less effort through a painful arc in the range of motion, yet still have high resistance in other areas in the range of motion. (3) Exercises may be performed at fast, functional contractile velocities.

The development of isokinetic resistance exercise has allowed the use of lower resistances and higher repetitions, resulting in better strength development and less joint trauma when high loads are avoided [15]. On the negative side, availability of isokinetic equipment is limited in some situations because of cost. Also, its use can become a time-consuming endeavor when multiple muscle groups must be exercised.

Cardiovascular Endurance

During the early phases of rehabilitation, an effort should be made to limit the loss of cardiovascular endurance. Since cardiovascular endurance is lost rapidly with cessation of training, any form of exercise that the athlete can engage in without further aggravating the injury should be encouraged [16].

Selection of a cardiovascular conditioning program for the latter stages of rehabilitation should be sports-specific; however, activities for the earlier stages should accommodate the injury. Stationary cycling is an excellent form of cardiovascular exercise. The unique advantage of this modality is that it may be used even when one leg is immobilized. Some models will allow for variation in workload and speed to provide a good anaerobic and aerobic workout.

Pool running allows for aerobic conditioning while providing a relatively weightless environment [16]. This is accomplished by having the athlete run in chest-high water. Pool running is particularly useful in lower extremity injuries in which impact loading should be minimized.

Psychological Aspects of Rehabilitation

A comprehensive rehabilitation program promotes a positive state of mind which will facilitate the physical reconditioning process. Rehabilitation is 75% psychological and 25% physiological. These are important considerations when dealing with the delicate psyche of the young athlete.

The athlete's physical condition and ability to perform in his/her chosen sport are intimately tied to a sense of well-being [17]. An injury that prevents the athlete from competing may be a devastating problem. Rehabilitation should be expedited to return the athlete to the sport as soon as is safely possible.

Faris [17] has proposed a format for addressing the psychological aspects of athletic rehabilitation. Phase I – Information is gathered about the patient and the injury, and rapport is established. In doing so, trust is earned and anxiety is reduced. Phase II – The nature of the injury and the rehabilitation process is explained to the patient. The stage is set for the patient to have a proper frame of mind about the rehabilitation process. Phase III – The patient's emotional reactions to the injury and treatment are addressed. Fear, anger and depression are normal responses. Phase IV – The patient is trained to perform rehabilitation exercises properly to maximize benefits.

Pressure and anxiety may mount in the athlete attempting to recover from injury. Much of it may arise from uncertainty and fear of failure. Nideffer [18] has pointed out how increasing pressure and anxiety may incite certain physiological responses (increased heart rate, blood pressure and muscle tension) and psychological responses (loss of concentration) that may interact to complicate the process of recovery. These problems, if recognized early, often respond to reassurance. However, in some cases referral to a psychological specialist may be necessary. Techniques such as biofeedback, progressive relaxation and attention control may be effective in alleviating these problems [18].

Conclusion

Comprehensive sports injury rehabilitation requires a team approach. An understanding of how musculoskeletal injury inpacts on other organ systems is necessary. Traditional rehabilitation techniques to restore strength, flexibility and endurance should be augmented with a graded program to reacclimate the athlete to the demands of the sport. The psychological aspects of rehabilitation should not be ignored, as they often impact on recovery.

References

1 Nicholas JA, Hershman EB: The Lower Extremity and Spine in Sports Medicine. St Louis, Mosby, 1986.
2 Knight KL: Guidelines for rehabilitation of sports injuries. Clin Sports Med 1985;4:405–416.
3 Marino M: Current concepts on rehabilitation in sports medicine; in Nicholas JA, Hershman ED (eds): The Lower Extremity and Spine in Sports Medicine. St Louis, Mosby, 1986, vol 1, pp 117–194.
4 Kegerreis S: The construction and implementation of functional progressions as a component of athletic rehabilitation. J Orthop Sports Phys Ther 1983;5:14–19.
5 Nicholas JA: Review and update on the progress of rehabilitation; in Hunter LY, Funk FJ (eds): Rehabilitation of the Injured Knee. St Louis, Mosby, 1984, pp 3–5.
6 Dehne E, Torp RP: Treatment of joint injuries by immediate mobilization. Clin Orthop 1971;77:218–231.
7 Sealy DG: Practical considerations in flexibility exercises for knee and lower extremity; in Hunter LY, Funk FJ (eds): Rehabilitation of the Injured Knee. St Louis, Mosby, 1984, pp 319–321.
8 Stover CN: Physical conditioning of the immature athlete. Orthop Clin 1987;13:525–540.

9 Surburg PR: Neuromuscular facilitation techniques in sports medicine. Phys Sportsmed 1981;9:115–126.
10 Delorme TL: Restoration of muscle power by heavy resistance exercises. J Bone Joint Surg 1945;22:645.
11 Rians CB, Weltman A, et al: Strength training for prepubescent male: Is it safe? Am J Sports Med 1987;15:483–489.
12 Smith MJ: Muscle fiber types: Their relationship to athletic training and rehabilitation. Orthop Clin 1983;14:403–411.
13 Steadman JR: Rehabilitation of athletic injuries. Am J Sports Med 1979;7:147–149.
14 Davies GJ: A Compendium of Isokinetic in Clinical Usage. New York, LaCrosse, S & S Publishers, 1984.
15 Dickinson A, Bennett KM: Therapeutic exercise. Clin Sports Med 1985;4:417–429.
16 Spain J: Prehabilitation. Clin Sports Med 1985;4:575–585.
17 Faris G: Psychologic aspects of athletic rehabilitation. Clin Sports Med 1985;4:545–552.
18 Nideffer RM: The injured athlete: Psychological factors in treatment. Orthop Clin 1983;14:373–385.

Received: June 21, 1989

James A. Nicholas, MD
Department of Orthopaedic Surgery
Lenox Hill Hospital
130 East 77th Street
New York, NY 10021 (USA)

Pediatrician 1990;17:267–277

0300–1245/90/0174–0267$2.75/0

Pediatric Physical Therapy in a Rehabilitation Setting

Heidi Eigsti, Marybeth Aretz, Lou Shannon

The Children's Hospital, Denver, Colo., USA

Key Words. Pain management · Range of motion · Muscle tone · Motor skills · Adaptive equipment training

Abstract. Pediatric rehabilitation is a rapidly growing field. Managing the pediatric patient requires experience and the appreciation of the contributions of health, social and educational professionals: physician, nurse, occupational therapist, learning specialist, recreational therapist, psychologist, social worker, and physical therapist. The responsibility of this multidisciplinary team is to assist the family and the child in attaining the highest realistic physical independence, to prevent musculoskeletal deformity and, therefore, to improve the overall quality of life. Successful rehabilitation will depend on the degree to which each professional considers the whole child when working to alleviate specific handicaps. The long-term rehabilitation of the pediatric patient is a joint team-family responsibility, and for treatment to be translated into daily life, full cooperation and commitment from the family is crucial. The physician is the coordinator of the rehabilitation team and is responsible for the initial assessment and diagnosis from which the team undertakes appropriate management. Ideally, the physician and team members communicate frequently to ensure congruent goals of treatment. The role of the physical therapist in the management of the pediatric rehabilitation patient relates to classifications of diagnosis. The authors present this guide to families and health professionals for using physical therapy resources.

Introduction

The multiple roles of physical therapy will be discussed for children with diagnoses of cerebral palsy (CP), high-risk infants, developmental delay, Down syndrome, mental retardation, head injury, spina bifida, spinal cord injury, skeletal disorders, chronic diseases, joint and connective tissue diseases, burns, and amputations.

Cerebral Palsy

CP is a global term for various kinds of non-progressive central nervous system (CNS) damage of diverse etiology. Although there are many clinical manifestations, the principles of treatment remain the same. Physical therapy serves to lessen the abnormal effect of the damaged CNS and to promote more normal movement patterns. Treatment techniques have been pioneered that treat the neurological manifestations of CP. In the forefront is neurodevelopmental treatment, or NDT. Created by Berta Bobath, physical therapist, and explained by Dr. Karel Bobath, neurophysiologist, this technique, simply stated, seeks to change the abnormal tone and to facilitate the normal movement patterns via righting and equilibrium reactions. A physical therapist with this specialized knowledge is trained in the development and analysis of normal and abnormal movements. In working with a child with absolute or questionable CP, the physical therapist studies the quality in which a child moves and analyzes the reason for this movement. With this knowledge, the NDT-trained therapist can use various treatment techniques to raise or lower abnormal muscle tone to a more normalized state. The therapist can then facilitate normal movement transitions using righting and equilibrium reactions and normal muscle synergies. Depending on the degree of involvement, the therapist may passively bring or minimally guide the child through a movement pattern to the sensorimotor experience of what is 'normal'. With repetition (though always slightly altered so it never becomes rote), the therapist lightens the guide of the hands so that the child becomes more active in his or her own movement. Because the abnormal is constantly being inhibited, the normal has a chance to emerge. Neurologically, this sets up the neural pathways in the brain that become the path of least resistance.

Early intervention for infants with CP or those who are detected as being at risk for development delay is a logical perspective of NDT. Compared to an older child where therapy focuses on already established abnormal postures, motor patterns and sensory experiences that must be changed, therapy for an infant can be directed toward facilitation of normal movement before the abnormal has a chance to be ingrained in the CNS.

Treatment doesn't end when a therapy session is finished. Crucial to this therapeutic philosophy is parent education. The physical therapist teaches the parent(s) ways to best carry, diaper, (un)dress, position, and handle the child so that abnormal postures and sensorimotor experiences are avoided and more normal sensorimotor experiences are provided. With parental involvement, repetition of the normal is even greater, the path of least resistance stronger, and the carry-over into daily life more likely. Play activities can also be recommended to further encourage or reinforce more normal movement.

The role of the physical therapist is not a solitary one in the management of CP; there are many 'team' members. The physical therapist may or may not receive the initial referral from a physician to see a child (depending on individual state regulations). Regardless, the doctor and therapist need to communicate regularly regarding the particular child's development, both normal and abnormal. When surgical intervention is being considered, the therapist can offer valuable information regarding present muscle function that may influence surgery outcome. Following surgery, the therapy focus, schedule and goals may change. Orthotic considerations also should be discussed by the physician and physical therapist, with close involvement of the orthotist. There are many types of orthotics with special adaptations which function to improve ankle, knee, and hip stability, inhibit hypertonicity, alter abnormal gait, and improve skeletal alignment. Adaptive equipment, such as wheelchairs, walkers, and bath equipment, can help the child with CP reach a higher level of independence. The physical therapist can offer information regarding the child's wheelchair access capabilities, seating difficulties and overall muscle function to assist the physician in ordering the best equipment options. When other disciplines are involved (i.e. occupational, speech), regular contact should be maintained to coordinate short- and long-term goals and to assist in reinforcing the various therapeutic efforts.

Since a child spends a large portion of the day at school, physical therapy continues in this setting. Often a school system has its own therapists and the rehabilitation physical therapist can coordinate therapeutic efforts by communicating with the school therapist. If school therapists are not available, the physical therapist can then work through the classroom teacher and/or aides, emphasizing special positioning, equipment, and desirable activity considerations.

Other Neurological Impairments

Neurological conditions such as muscular neuropathies, meningitis, muscular dystrophy, and brain tumors often result in clinical manifestations affecting gross motor development. Therapy goals for these children are to restore normal range of motion, muscle strength and to help them reach their full gross motor potential. The physical therapist can employ the same NDT philosophy and treatment strategies as used in treating CP. Often, these patients have coordination problems as well as balance and equilibrium difficulties. The therapist has special treatment tools to facilitate improved performance in these areas. When working with a Guillain-Barré patient, care is taken to work only within the child's limits. Muscle fatigue is avoided as this can hinder restoration of normal muscle strength.

For children with muscular dystrophy, or any other dystrophy, goals again focus on improving range of motion, strength and gross motor function. A physical therapist works with the child and family to keep the patient ambulating for as long as possible. Once ambulation is no longer feasible, the therapist determines equipment needs and training for mobility and daily living skills.

High-Risk Infants

Increased survival rates for infants with a low birth weight and infants with major medical problems have raised an interest in initiating developmentally appropriate care to infants in newborn and special-care nurseries. These infants often remain medically fragile with respiratory and cardiovascular compromise, tracheostomy and gastrostomy tubes, seizure disorders, and other severe neurologic damage [1]. Low birth weight and premature infants are generally at higher risk for developmental delay and handicapping conditions. Although questions still exist as to what kinds of stimulation should be provided, enough research has been conducted to institute Public Law 99-457 which mandates the provision of services to this high-risk group.

The programs for high-risk infants are based on the belief that the first years of life are critical for intervention because of the plasticity of the CNS and the rapid developmental changes. The purpose of these programs is to provide support and training to parents in understanding the developmental needs of their infant and to provide continuity of developmental support both in the hospital and after discharge.

The physical therapist performs a neuromotor evaluation to assess the infant's reflex development, postural responses, range of motion, muscle tone, response to handling, and appropriateness of physical therapy intervention. There are many evaluation tools available for this purpose. The Morgan neonatal neurobehavioral examination is frequently used for the term or preterm infant [2]. Ellison's infant neurological international battery is available for the older infant [3]. Als' *Assessment of Premature Infant Behavior* documents the infant's response to stimulation, ability to quiet himself and smoothness of change in behavioral states [4]. The Dubowitz's *Neurological Assessment of the Pre-Term and Full-Term Infant* looks at tone, reflexes and behavioral responses [5]. Ameil-Teison has two books on infant evaluation: *Neurologic Evaluation of the Newborn* [6] and the *Infant and Neurologic Assessment during the First Year of Life* [7]. The reader is referred to *Neurological Development in the Fullterm and Premature Neonate* [8] and to the discussion of neurodevelopmental symptoms during the first year of life [9] for further description of early behavior and development. Chandler's manual, *Movement Assessment in Infants* [10], is also a valuable reference. Following the evaluation, specific treatment strategies for positioning and handling are developed. This planning requires a sound knowledge of normal and abnormal development as well as the influences of primitive reflexes. Handling techniques are based on the NDT approach and are modified for the infant's age and medical status. Positioning is very important to inhibit abnormal tone and facilitate normal development and must be adapted to accommodate for medical equipment such as ventilator, intubation, tracheostomy and gastrostomy tubes, heart monitors, ileostomies, and IV sites. The parent is the key interventionist and must be educated in handling, positioning and intervention skills.

Developmental Delays

Etiologies of a developmental delay are many: mental retardation, understimulation, chronic illness, and visual deficits are a few. The diagnosis of delayed development requires a complete evaluation of motor skills, speech, vision, behavior, and cognition. Children with suspected delays are often referred to physical therapy for a thorough assessment of motor development as well as recommendations for physical therapy intervention.

There are a number of standardized tests available which provide objective measures for assessing developmental age-equivalent levels. Although helpful, these tests do not objectively measure the quality of the child's movement, muscle tone, strength, posture, range of motion, or flexibility. These components also must be evaluated by the physical therapist. Following evaluation, a treatment plan is devised based on the principles of NDT. The mode of delivery and the functional goals are adjusted according to the child's developmental stage. Therapy sessions generally incorporate exercise into functional play activities to correct specific weaknesses of the individual child. The program also educates the parents to structure the child's activities and to provide an optimal learning environment. Success of treatment depends largely upon the extent of the delay, parent involvement, and cooperation from the child.

Down Syndrome, Mental Retardation

Children with Down syndrome or other various forms of mental retardation can possess postural deficiencies and experience movement disturbances. They tend to have varying degrees of hypotonia, along with ligamentous laxity and diminished proximal joint stability; decreased ability for graded, mid-range control during movement results. Often 'fixing' or excessive holding in compensatory muscle groups occurs, which interferes with normal movement patterns and the development of equilibrium reactions. A physical therapist can therapeutically alter a child's muscle tone, posture and movement patterns to help prevent future skeletal deformity, joint/muscle contractures and inefficient movement patterns.

Children with Down syndrome and mentally retarded children with hypotonicity problems often receive physical therapy in the school setting rather than in a hospital or center-based setting. This is most appropriate, as therapeutic intervention can be incorporated into functional classroom activities and daily living skills. The physical therapist changes the techniques and activities used to accommodate the child's level of cognitive functioning and understanding.

Hypotonicity is 'the root of all evil' because it leads to other subsequent problems, primarily orthopedic concerns and impaired balance and equilibrium. The therapist focuses the treatment on specific problems the individual child demonstrates. One general goal is to increase overall muscle tone. Increasing antigravity (postural) strength must be addressed, via appropriate extension activities, to prevent or minimize kyphosis. Rectus and oblique abdominal muscles must be strengthened. This will help support the viscera of the abdominal cavity which will, in turn, help support the lumbar spine as well as pull the pelvis in a posterior tilt and decrease the lumbar lordosis. Obtaining good hip abductor strength plays a key role in preventing hip subluxation/dislocation. Knee recurvatum is common in hypotonic children. Increasing proximal control, correcting an anteriorly tilted pelvis and increasing the strength of the quadriceps and hamstrings help remedy this problem. Ankle and foot alignment is also a prime concern for these children. Pronation with calcaneal valgus is common. This malalignment influences the skeletal alignment above, further encouraging knee recurvatum, hip flexion, anterior pelvic tilt, and lumbar lordosis. Orthotics may be prescribed to realign the calcaneus with the talus and tibia and possibly affect skeletal alignment. Atlanto-axial malalignment is also common in Down syndrome, secondary to ligamentous laxity and/or congenital anomaly of the C1-C2 vertebrae. This abnormality can be detected by x-ray and should be routinely checked before a child enters school or begins any type of gross motor/movement therapy. Any abnormal x-ray finding must be relayed to the physical therapist so that certain therapeutic activities can be modified or avoided completely.

Mentally retarded children who are affected more severely (having very low cognitive function and movement abilities secondary to severe spasticity or hypotonia) require a different focus by the physical therapist. Goals for these children address positioning in bed as well as in various pieces of equipment (i.e. sidelyers and special seating devices) to help prevent contractures. General stimulation techniques can be employed. Recommending, ordering, and adapting special equipment becomes a top priority of the treating therapist. Use of standers, prone or supine, is controversial at this point as they are purely passive and benefits are unproven. The physical therapist should be aware of the pros and cons of their use and choose to use them cautiously for specific purposes for short periods of time.

Traumatic Head Injury

Childhood head injuries are often caused by impression from blunt trauma, shear from acceleration and hemorrhage from whiplash (shake). Damage is generally irreversible but may be reduced with treatment, although rehabilitation for these children is often costly and extensive. These children often are impaired in vision, hearing, speech, fine motor tasks, cognition, and gross motor development and, therefore, must be managed by a multidisciplinary team. Deficits depend on the mechanism and location of the injury.

Multisensory stimulation for coma patients includes vestibular, kinesthetic, tactile, auditory, proprioceptive, and visual stimuli. Exercises to maintain a range of motion are begun early and continued throughout the rehabilitation process.

Often the CNS damage is manifested as abnormal tone and movement. It is the therapist's role to use handling techniques, positioning and splinting to inhibit abnormal tone and facilitate normal movement patterns. Neurodevelopmental techniques are used to achieve appropriate gross motor skills.

Adaptive equipment such as wheelchairs, walkers and braces are commonly employed to improve the overall level of independence. The physical therapist educates the child and family on the proper use of this equipment and consults in home modification planning.

Fortunately, children have greater potential for recovery after head trauma than adults, and improvement is likely to continue up to 5 years posttrauma. Most children need ongoing therapy for motor disorders with anticipation of changes due to growth. Outpatient physical therapy management of children with head injuries is very similar to the management of children with cerebral palsy and is based on the NDT approach.

Spina Bifida

Spina bifida is a common congenital abnormality characterized by the incomplete closure of one or more neural arches [11]. Classifications are determined by the amount of separation of the vertebral elements at the midline and the amount of neural tube involvement. The most common classifications are occult, manifesta and aperta.

Children with spina bifida require care by a multidisciplinary team consisting of a neurosurgeon, pediatrician, orthopedist, urologist, physiatrist, occupational and physical therapist. The objectives of the physical therapist are to minimize contractures and spinal deformity and to assist the child in normal development.

The most common lesions occur in the lumbosacral region. Neurological deficits are most often found in the lower extremities and vary from mild muscle imbalance and sensory loss to complete paraplegia. The most common deformities caused by muscle imbalance and/or paralysis are hip dislocations, knee contractures and foot deformities.

Hip dislocation frequently results from unopposed hip flexors. Unilateral dislocation is always treated; however, there is much controversy as to whether bilateral dislocation should be treated. Conservative treatment includes traction, casting and the use of prone standers. The therapist is responsible for the size adjustments and time schedule for prone stander activities and for training the parents in the use of the stander. Surgical intervention is another treatment option available for hip dislocation. Knee flexion contractures develop when hamstring spasticity exists in combination with weak or absent quadricep function. Contractures also may occur in children who have flaccid hamstrings or quadriceps, and who do not receive physical therapy for passive range of motion. The key to management of knee contractures is daily hamstring stretching performed by the parent. Strengthening of the quadriceps is equally important to provide hamstring opposition. In more severe cases, surgical procedures are required to lengthen the hamstrings. Physical therapy following hamstring lengthening is essential to maintain a range of motion and to assist the child in strengthening the proper muscles.

Equinovarus, calcaneovalgus, vertical talus, pes cavus, and ankle valgus are common deformities seen with spina bifida. Mild conditions can be treated with conservative methods such as stretching, selective muscle strengthening and casting by a physical therapist well trained in proper foot alignment. More severe cases often require surgical intervention. Postsurgical physical therapy is critical in maintaining proper foot alignment and in selecting appropriate orthotics, casts or braces. Kyphosis and scoliosis are the two most frequent spinal deformities in children with spina bifida. These conditions may be congenital or may be associated with vertebral body abnormalities or weakness of the dorsal musculature. Mild conditions are managed through exercise or use of a Milwaukee brace. Larger curves may require surgical intervention.

Various types of adaptive equipment and orthotics can promote normal development in children with spina bifida, as seen in figure 1.

The physical therapist is responsible for training the parents and child in the proper use of these devices and for monitoring skin integrity and proper fit of equipment. Many children with spina bifida use wheelchairs for mobility. Wheelchair training for independence is incorporated into the child's physical therapy sessions. The overall goal for these children is to make them as functionally independent as possible while minimizing musculoskeletal deformities.

Spinal Cord Injuries

The incidence of childhood traumatic spinal cord injury increases with age [13]. The primary causes of spinal cord injury in children are motor vehicle accidents and auto-pedestrian accidents. Falls and sports injuries are the second most common cause. The time and money invested in these children's rehabilitation is extensive; the mean period of hospital stay is 3–5 months, depending on the level of involvement. The physical therapist is responsible for evaluation, treatment and management of multiple aspects of rehabilitation in spinal cord injury. During the initial evaluation, the physical therapist assesses muscle strength and substitution through careful manual muscle testing to determine the potential level of independence. This examination sets the goals of the rehabilitation process, training and equipment needs.

Skin integrity and lack of sensation directly affect postures and positions available during treatment; skin breakdown results in training delays and increased hospital stays if prevention measures such as weightshifts and positioning are not initiated by the physical therapist. The therapist educates the family, patient and staff in the proper care of skin over bony prominence and scar

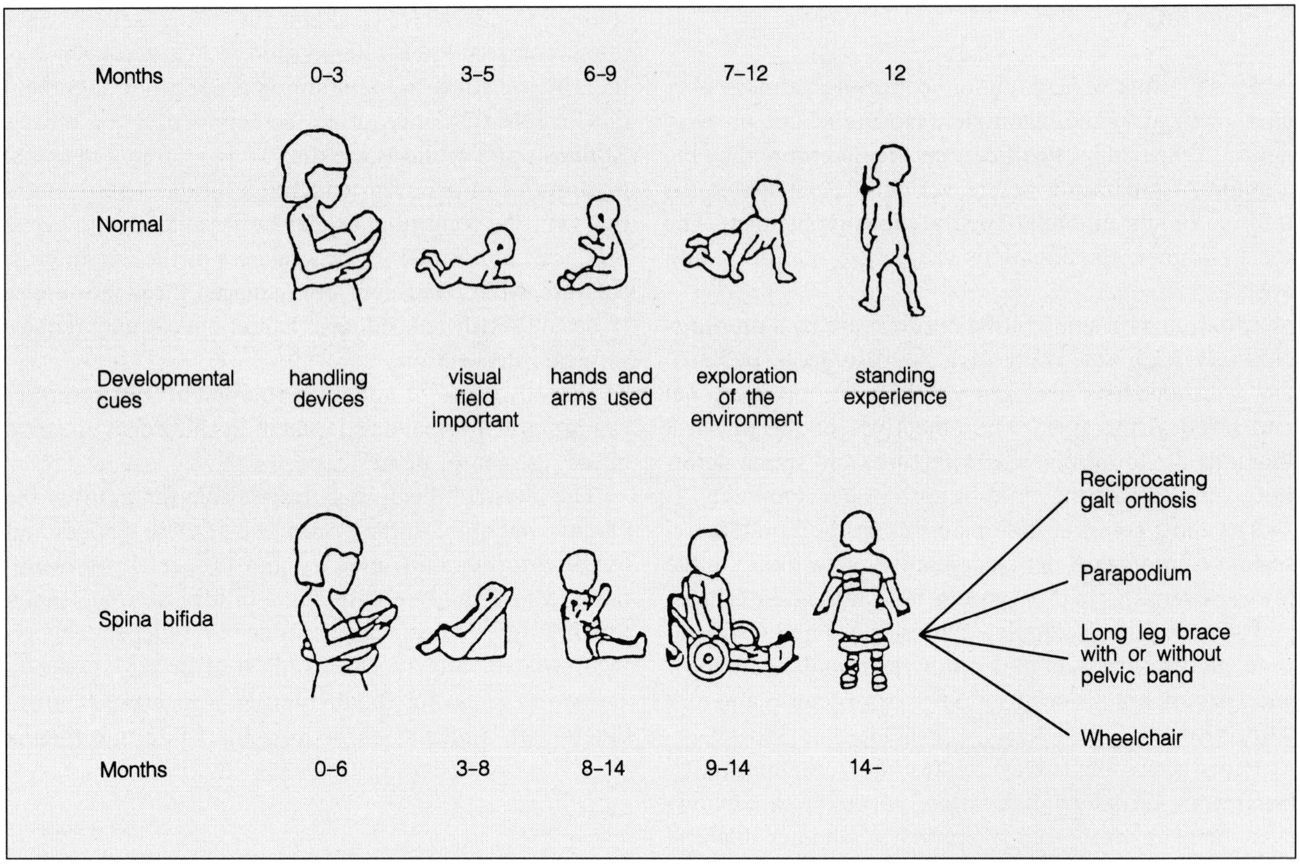

Fig. 1. Orthotic devices for the child with moderate spina bifida at progressive stages of development and ages, compared with crawling and standing of normal child. Child begins sitting stage with assistance of caster cart, uses reciprocating gait orthosis for standing and walking. Children aged 17 months to 14 years who have flaccid paralysis can wear a parapodium to facilitate rolling, standing from a prone position, and swivel walking. By the age of 10 years, many children will prefer the use of a wheelchair when walking becomes too energy consuming [12]. (With permission [16].)

tissue breakdown. Timely weight shifts and adequate cushions can relieve pressure on the ischials and sacrum.

Deficits in sensation due to lack of sensory feedback may impair coordination, making motor skills, self-care and activities of daily living more difficult to master. The therapist evaluates all sensory receptors, pain, temperature, touch, and proprioception. A treatment plan is then designed to increase the child's awareness and ability to compensate for these deficits.

If the spinal cord is transected above C3 level, innervation of the phrenic nerve and, thus, the ability to initiate inspiration are lost [14]. These children require artificial life support systems (artificial ventilation, phrenic stimulation). If the cord is transected below C3, the ability to inspire is present, but good expiration may be lacking if abdominal muscle strength and tone are affected. Good breathing skills must be taught to be coordinated with functional activities to improve endurance and skill in operating sip and puff controls. Passive manual stretches and joint mobilization techniques can be applied to the chest wall to promote trunk range of motion. With the assistance of respiratory therapy, games may be included in treatment to improve respiratory muscle strength.

Extremes in joint range (i.e. low back, hamstrings, long finger flexors) often play an important role in compensating for strength deficits. The therapist provides the child and family with a program to incorporate full range of motion and selective lengthening. This promotes optimal independence with transfers and activities of daily living.

In lower motor neuron lesions, muscle tone tends to increase the first 2 years following the injury. Some children can learn to use this tone for functional purposes. More often, however, the therapist must assist in positioning techniques to inhibit this tone to maintain good joint alignment, prevent contractures and skin breakdown.

Often children with spinal cord injuries have a poor tolerance for vertical positioning. The physical therapist monitors the patient's blood pressure, pulse and pallor while gradually raising the patient's vertical position in bed. Once the patient can tolerate getting out of bed, work on transfers, endurance, coordination, balance, gait (depending on level of lesion), and wheel chair mobility can begin. The child must be trained to be as independent as possible on all types of terrain. The therapist teaches the child to overcome unexpected circumstances such as inaccessible buildings and stairs. The child should be able to instruct any caretaker in assisting with transfers and wheelchair mobility as appropriate.

Rehabilitation is also the time to prepare the family and patient for discharge. Often modifications are necessary to make the home accessible to wheelchairs. The therapist can assist the family in the planning of these modifications and in the ordering of any special equipment (bathseats, Hoyer lifts, electric and manual wheelchairs, vans, and van lifts).

Once the child returns home, the second phase of rehabilitation begins. For the paraplegic, this may include endurance training with adaptive equipment. For the quadriplegic it may mean wheelchair mobility. When the child reaches maximum rehabilitation potential, long-term monitoring continues to decrease chances of scoliosis, spinal deformity, hip dislocation, pelvic obliquities, skin breakdown, and inadequate wheelchair or orthotic fit.

Orthopedic Rehabilitation

The term 'orthopedics' covers a broad spectrum, and the role the physical therapist plays in this area is a varied one. General goals are to provide clinical findings to the physician, to restore or improve joint range of motion and muscle strength, to train patients in the use of adaptive equipment, and to correct gait deviations – all to improve overall daily functioning and independence.

The manner in which a physical therapist manages a special orthopedic problem is dependent on the presenting problem. This section will attempt to describe the role of the physical therapist by grouping similar orthopedic diagnoses and describing the general points of treatment.

Skeletal disorders include many varied diagnoses ranging from arthrogryposis to congenital hip dislocation. In therapy, passive and active range of motion of the involved joint(s), stretching of the surrounding shortened musculature, and strengthening exercises are implemented. The patient (if old enough) and/or family is instructed in a home program complimenting activities in therapy. Splints worn during the day or only at night may be needed to provide proper positioning and to provide a maintained passive stretch to elongate tightened muscle and soft tissue. Serial casting may be necessary, especially for the arthrogrypotic child, where joint contractures are severe and the range of motion is grossly limited. Orthotics may be prescribed to correct and maintain proper tibial-ankle-foot alignment or to compensate for weakness at the ankle joint. Surgical intervention often is required in children with skeletal disorders. Here, the physical therapist will continue efforts to restore the full range of motion and muscle strength and to aid the child in restoring or, in more severe cases, maximizing his/her potential for gross motor independence and ambulation.

Length discrepancies of the lower extremity, as seen in skeletal length deficiency, Legg-Calvé-Perthes disease, or congenitally dislocated hip cause an inefficient gait pattern. For discrepancies of 1.5–3 cm in leg length, a shoe lift of appropriate height may be all that is needed. For differences of 3–6 cm a surgical correction may be required. In this case, the therapist is available post-surgically to restore the joint range. If pain is an inhibiting factor for a child attempting to exercise on the range of motion and strength, the therapist may try a transcutaneous electrical nerve stimulation unit to help diminish the discomfort at rest and with activity. Weakened musculature can be strengthened by a variety of methods – isometric, traditional concentric/eccentric, and by functional upright activities. An electrical stimulation unit may be used to prevent atrophy, enhance muscle strength or for muscle reeducation.

Transfer training may initially be necessary in the acute phase. Ambulation training, with or without an assistive device, includes negotiation of stairs and uneven terrain. Rehabilitation can also be targeted at specific gait problems to improve the quality of ambulation. Bracing or orthotics may be necessary and the physical therapist can offer knowledge and assistance in the recommendation, fitting and functional use of these devices.

Physical therapy is involved in the areas of chronic pain as seen with chondromalacia, Osgood-Schlatter disease, general musculo-skeletal pain, tendinitis, and other forms of overuse syndromes and sports injuries in the adolescent patient. Regardless of the degree of insult, the goals of physical therapy remain true to orthopedic rehabilitation: to relieve pain via modalities, to restore the full range of motion, to increase strength, to improve gross motor function, and to develop a normal gait pattern. The therapist is also responsible for educating the patient regarding the kinds of athletic or general activities to avoid or prevent further injury.

Postural disorders treated by a physical therapist vary from scoliosis to low back pain secondary to poor postural habits. An evaluation is performed to create a treatment program addressing the primary problems. Therapy involves patient education regarding proper posture and body mechanics, and selective stretching and strengthening exercises usually given in the form of a home program. Regular and appropriately timed rechecks are scheduled and progress is documented. Any concerns experienced by the physical therapist are relayed to the treating physician.

Prevention is the 'buzz' word in the field of orthopedic physical therapy. Here, the physical therapist plays the role of an educator to help reduce the risk of injury, instructing clients in body mechanics, joint protection, hazards of overuse, and stretching.

Chronic Respiratory Disease

Chronic respiratory diseases frequently seen in children are asthma, cystic fibrosis, and bronchopulmonary dysplasia. When breathing becomes difficult, these children often assume a habitual flexed posture of spinal kyphosis, chest contraction, elevated and protracted shoulders and scapulae, and a forward-leaning head. Depending on the severity of the disease, children may also adopt an inactive lifestyle. The global goal of a physical therapist working in the area of respiratory diseases is to keep these patients mobile and as active as possible to prevent respiratory infections. The treating therapist must be sensitive to the child's capabilities and must individualize the treatment program to the limitations of each child.

The role of the therapist working with children with respiratory disorders depends on the established departmental policies of the healthcare facility. At some locations, percussion and vibration is a physical therapy inpatient responsibility; in others, it is the respiratory therapist's. If the latter is true, the physical therapist collaborates with the respiratory therapist to reinforce any relaxation and/or breathing techniques performed during therapy and at rest. The choice of more traditional treatment activities depends on whether the child is ventilator-dependent or is able to move freely within the environment. For ventilator-dependent patients, the therapist focuses on the prevention of joint contractures. This is achieved via passive and active range of motion techniques. Proper bed positioning also is necessary, and the therapist educates the nursing staff, the patient (if appropriate), and parents in this skill. Increasing and maintaining muscle strength is important for motoric function, mobility and transitional movement purposes. Isometrics and various traditional strengthening exercises using weights or resistance are employed. Mobility and function can be achieved through activities such as rolling and transitional movements. For children with severe respiratory distress transfer training may be necessary, as this activity, in itself, may be an extremely frightening and threatening experience. If the use of a portable ventilator is possible, then ambulation and independent wheelchair mobility skills may become a desirable goal.

For children who are independent of a ventilator, flexibility and prevention of extremity joint contractures are also important. Strengthening and increasing overall endurance can be accomplished with traditional exercise, bicycle riding, use of the treadmill or rowing machine, or can be incorporated into creative therapeutic activities. Sensitivity to a child's limits and regular monitoring of heart rate, blood pressure and respiratory rate are essential during exercise. Postural exercises may be prescribed to strengthen anti-gravity musculature, to assist in expanding the chest cavity for improved lung function and to re-educate the child to maintain a more normal posture.

Joint and Connective Tissue Disease

Medical management of the child with juvenile rheumatoid arthritis requires a multidisciplinary team. The main objectives are to reduce inflammation, preserve function and prevent deformity. Ideally, this will lead to optimal independence in physical, psychological, vocational, and educational functions.

In the acute phase, the child is ill with fever and a variety of systemic symptoms. At this point, the physical therapist is active as a consultant for good positioning, splinting and gentle range of motion in the pain-free range. Modalities such as superficial heat (hot pack, ultrasound, whirlpool, and paraffin) may help in pain relief. Exercise for maintenance and improvement of muscle strength, with emphasis on isometric and active assistive range of motion, is given as the child's condition improves. Functional and recreational activities with minimum joint stress (such as swimming) are encouraged. The therapist also assesses the child's needs for assistive aids to improve overall independence. Wheelchairs, walkers and canes may improve self reliance and thus reduce personal and family stress.

Burns

Only a well organized multidisciplinary team can provide optimal rehabilitation for the burned child. The objectives of the physical therapist are to prevent burn wound sepsis, promote proper healing, minimize secondary deformities and hypertrophic scarring, prevent postural and gait abnormalities, and prevent regression of motor development. The timing and extent of physical therapy involvement is directed by the physician.

The potential for contracture and functional impairment is greatest when the wound approximates joints or body creases [15]. Prevention of this complication is accomplished by passive and active range of motion. When performed while the child is submerged in the whirlpool, it is generally less painful. Range of motion is also performed outside the whirlpool, while the patient is wearing dressings, to assure the maintenance of range of motion between baths. Stretching maintains and lengthens scar tissue on healed burns, and paraffin wax application and ultrasound are often beneficial for the combined effects of heat, lubrication and softening. Deep massage of scar tissue promotes softening and further lengthening. The therapist avoids extreme or sudden range of motion as this may tear healing tissue or cause bleeding. The exercises are performed gently when the burn extends through muscle or tendon or where there is an electric burn of unknown depth. The child is encouraged to assist with range of motion exercises as able to prepare for ambulation.

Ambulation is a major tool in counteracting the debilitating effects of immobility/venous stasis, contracture and loss of strength [14]. Therefore, the child is assisted with ambulation as soon as possible after transfer from the ICU. The child's lower extremities are wrapped in ace bandages prior to ambulation to prevent swelling. Therapists use age-appropriate developmental tasks for stretching and strengthening of selective muscles, as well as to encourage progression of normal motor development. This encourages independence and improves the child's psychological attitude. Positioning is designed to oppose the forces and patterns of wound contracture. The nursing staff and family are instructed in positioning programs designed by the therapist and the child is placed in a variety of positions throughout the day.

Splinting is frequently necessary when the child cannot achieve full range of motion, when the child consistently holds the joint in a contracture pattern, when pressure is needed to minimize hypertrophic scarring, or to aid in contouring of the face, neck and chin. Splints produce hard nonyielding pressure which softens and flattens scars. They may be worn by the patient at all times or only at night, depending on individual needs, and are always removed for exercises. Children are frequently candidates for splinting because of their noncompliance with positioning. The physical therapist measures, fits, and monitors pressure garments used for healed burned areas if there are signs of hypertrophic scar development or if an area sustained a deep partial or full thickness burn. The skin is prepared for pressure garments by desensitization measures using elastic bandage and tubular bandage to build up tolerance. Continuous pressure produces a more organized configuration of collagen bundles yielding a flatter, softer scar that matures more rapidly.

Hospital discharge signals the successful completion of one stage of rehabilitation and the beginning of another. These children require regular follow-up with a multidisciplinary team to prevent secondary complications. They often continue physical therapy on an outpatient basis and the family is educated in a home program that incorporates stretching, massage, strengthening, and pressure garment wear.

Physical Therapy for Children with Limb Deficiencies

Children may be born with limb deficiencies or experience amputations through disease or accident. The cause of congenital limb deficiency is usually unknown, although some deficiencies have been reported in conjunction with certain syndromes.

The etiology of acquired amputations falls into three categories: (1) traumatic – resulting from accidents, burns or crushing injuries; (2) illness-related – necessitated by tumors or vascular problems, and (3) surgical revision – amputation of a deformed or nonfunctional limb.

The juvenile amputee is a challenge which is best met by a multi-disciplinary team with a common knowledge of children, their growth and development, and a dedicated patience to follow the child and family through the child's growing years. The child's pediatrician or family physician should be encouraged to work closely with the amputee team. This team may include an orthopedist, nurse, physiatrist, psychiatrist, psychologist, clinical social worker, a physical therapist, an occupational therapist, and a prosthetist with special training in fabricating and fitting prostheses for children. The child and his/her family or caretakers must be considered prime members of the rehabilitation team.

'Habilitation' and therapy for the congenital amputee begins the day the child is born. 'Rehabilitation' and subsequent therapy for the acquired amputee begins when a decision is made to amputate. The congenital and acquired amputee will require close follow-up from the team to address the problems associated with the psychosocial, psychological and musculoskeletal systems of the child. The family must understand the importance and role of each team member. The importance of the physician/clinic and physical therapist having good working relationships with the child and family must be stressed. All therapy sessions must include family participation to guarantee optimal care and training at home.

Generally, physical therapists treat children with absences of lower limbs and occupational therapists are responsible for treatment of absent upper limbs. However, therapists from both disciplines have a working knowledge of growth and development and can assess whether the child is performing within the normal range. The remainder of this article provides information related to the child with lower extremely deficiencies.

When the child is first referred for physical therapy, a preprosthetic evaluation is performed. This includes a developmental screening as well as measurements of bone lengths and circumferences, skin color and condition, scars, muscle bulk, sensation, and edema of the deficient side as compared to the sound side. Following the evaluation, a program of preprosthetic therapy is designed.

There are four major areas of treatment considered in the preprosthetic care of the juvenile amputee:

(1) stump shrinkage through proper ace bandaging or rigid dressing (light-weight cast); (2) reduction of contractures or tightness; (3) maintenance of normal range of motion, and (4) facilitation of normal developmental milestones and maximal strength.

The child (if old enough) and parents must become an integral part of the 'team'. The therapist instructs them in home exercises to be done at least twice a day until the prosthesis is received. Home exercise programs can often be incorporated into routine activities such as bathing and dressing. Prosthetic evaluation is conducted with the physician, therapist and prosthetist, all consulting together with the child and family. The lower extremity congenital amputee is fit with a prosthesis when the child begins to pull to stand. The acquired amputee is fit with a prosthesis as soon as the incision is healed and the stump has shrunk enough to tolerate and suspend a prosthesis.

There are many new developments in prosthetic design and materials with modern protheses being more functional, more cosmetically acceptable and lighter in weight than older devices. The chosen prosthesis is determined by age, the extent of limb deficiency, the condition of the stump, and the developmental or functional level of performance. To some extent the extreme cost of some prostheses may be a determining factor.

A prosthetic check-out on all new prostheses or on major changes in old prostheses is ideally performed jointly by the therapist and prosthetist. This evaluation consists of: (1) checking movable joints for quality materials and workmanship; (2) mechanical checking to determine alignment of trochanter, knee, ankle, and correct fitting of the socket, and (3) functional checking to ensure usability of prostheses during movement and activities (this may take several sessions until the child feels comfortable with the prosthesis).

Initial therapy sessions with the therapist and parent are intensive. For the very young child, therapy sessions are combined with play sessions, whereas the older child's therapy can coincide with functional sessions.

Goal setting is dependent upon age and severity of limb loss. The therapist sets goals with the parents for very young children; however, children who are 5 years old and older play an important part in setting their own goals.

The physical therapist's roles in rehabilitation include the assessment of various aspects of motor behavior and planning, and implementing programs to guide and facilitate motor and perceptual development. In addition to providing direct treatment services, the physical therapist provides consultative and indirect services to other disciplines.

Conclusion

Strategies for physical therapy treatment are specific for each diagnosis and are further individualized according to each child's needs. Physical therapy goals, however, can be broadly defined to include all diagnoses. In general, the physical therapist strives to decrease pain, to maximize joint range of motion, normalize muscle tone, to prevent musculoskeletal deformity, to improve strength and endurance, and to develop age-appropriate gross motor skills with or without the use of adaptive equipment. The physical therapist also serves to educate the family and is a continued support and resource for the child's future rehabilitation needs. The physical therapist works with other health care professionals to assist each child in reaching his/her maximum level of independence and to improve his/her quality of life.

References

1 Long, T.; Katz, K.; Pokorni, J.: Developmental intervention with the chronically ill infant. Infant young Child. *2:* 78 (1989).
2 Morgan, A.M.; Koch, V.; Aldag, J.: Neonatal neurobehavioral examination. A new instrument for quantitative analysis of neonatal neurological status. Phys. Ther. *68:* 1352–1358 (1988).
3 Ellison, P.; Horn, J.; Browning, O.: Construction of an infant neurological international battery (INFANIB) for the assessment of neurological integrity in infancy. Phys. Ther. *11:* 63–66 (1982).
4 Als, H.; Tronic, E.; Lester, B.M.: Manual for the assessment of pre-term infant's behavior (APIB); in Fitzgerald, Lester, Yogman (eds): Theory and research in behavioral pediatrics, vol. 1, pp. 63–133 (Plenum Press, New York 1982).
5 Dubowitz, V.; Dubowitz, L.: Neurological assessment of the preterm and full-term infant. (William Heimann Medical Books, London 1981).
6 Amiel-Tison, C.: Neurological evaluation of the newborn and the infant. (Masson, New York 1986).
7 Amiel-Tison, C.: Neurological assessment during the first year of life. (Oxford University Press, New York 1986).
8 Saint-Anne Dargassies, S.: Neurological development in the full-term and premature neonate. (Elsevier, Amsterdam 1977).
9 Saint-Anne Dargassies, S.: Neurodevelopmental symptoms during the first year of life. Part I. Essential landmarks for each key age. Devl. Med. Child Neur. *14:* 235–246 (1972).
10 Chandler, L.; Swanson, M.: Movement assessment in infants: a manual. (Roung Bay, Washington 1980).
11 Salter, B.: Spina bifida; in Curtiss, Textbook of disorders and injuries of the musculoskeletal system; 2nd ed., pp. 132–133 (Waverly Press, Baltimore 1983).
12 Motloch, W.: Orthotic philosophies of treatment. Clin. Prosthet. Orthot. *8:* 10 (1984).
13 Menkes, J.: Textbook of child neurology; 2nd ed. (Lea and Febiger, Philadelphia, 1979).
14 Nixon, V.: Respiration; in Schneider, Spinal cord injury; 1st ed. (Aspen Publishers, Salem, 1985).
15 Helm, P.; Kevorkian, A.; Lushbaugh, M.; et al.: Burn injury: rehabilitation management in 1982. J Burn Care Rehabil. *4:* 413 (1982).
16 Motloch, W.M.; Brearly, M.N.: Technical note – a patient-propelled variable-inclination prone stander. Prosthet. Orthotics int. *7:* 176–177 (1983).

Received: August 1, 1989

Heidi Eigsti
Physical Therapy Department
The Children's Hospital
1056 E. 19th Ave.
Denver, CO 80218 (USA)

Pediatrician 1990;17:278–282

0300–1245/90/0174–0278$2.75/0

Occupational Therapy in Pediatric Rehabilitation

Charlotte Brasic Royeen[a], *Delia Gorga*[b]

[a]Research and Therapy Services, Great Falls, Va.; [b]The New York Hospital, Cornell Medical Center, N.Y., USA

Key Words. Rehabilitation · Occupational therapy · Function

Abstract. Occupational therapy in pediatric rehabilitation focuses on the effects of diseases and of the environment on a child's abilities to function successfully in daily life settings (home, school and playground) and roles (family member, student, etc.). In this paper, the process of pediatric occupational therapy, from assessment to discharge planning, is briefly described. Pediatric occupational therapy intervention strategies including treatment, environmental adaptation, and systems change are presented and illustrated. Three case studies highlighting occupational therapy intervention are discussed.

Occupational therapists are concerned with disease or ill effects of the environment on the abilities or performance areas of infants and children (table 1) which interfere with the development or maintenance of meaningful roles (family member, student, playmate, etc.). Occupational therapists consider engagement in such roles to be occupations. In the infant with cerebral palsy, for example, the occupational therapist is concerned that the underlying pathology affects the infant's acquisition of functional mobility, self-maintenance, ability to calm self, and play related to the infant's occupational role development as family member and student. In the case of the child with a developmental delay with no known organic cause, the occupational therapist is concerned with environmental factors that inhibit or facilitate occupational role development. In this case, the occupational therapist may question: 'How is the child handled at home? Does the environment provide a variety of activities and social interactions? Is the child successfully interacting with the parent during feeding and play?'

The five largest pediatric groups served by occupational therapists are the developmentally delayed, children with cerebral palsy, the mentally retarded, children with adjustment disorders and those with affective disorders (table 2). The first two groups combined constitute approximately 78% of the patient population served by occupational therapists.

Criteria for Referral

How does one know when an infant or child should be referred to occupational therapy for screening and/or assessment? Patterns of problems leading to dysfunction in performance areas and resultant difficulties in role acquisition (occupation) are the criteria for referral. Table 3 presents referral criteria for occupational therapy services.

The Process of Occupational Therapy

Assessment

The pediatric occupational therapy process begins with assessment. Occupational therapy assessment includes, but is not limited to: (1) understanding the medical diagnosis and reason for referral; (2) obtaining the

Table 1. Performance areas with examples

Performance area	Examples
Functional mobility	use of hands for manipulation and exploration, ability to navigate space, for independence and need gratification
Self maintenance	feeding, dressing, grooming, toileting
Play	exploration of playground environments, use of toys
Regulatory processes	sleep/wake cycles, ability to filter out extraneous stimuli, ability to calm self
Educational readiness	visual perceptual ability, eye-hand coordination, ability to organize and sequence, ability to attend
Socialization	peer interactions, interaction with parents and siblings, response to authority
Emotional stability	ability to control self, development of delayed gratification, development of appropriate assertiveness

This chart has been adapted from concepts presented in Pratt and Allen [4] and the American Occupational Therapy Association's draft version of uniform terminology [5].

parental or guardian's (teacher or health care worker also as appropriate) views of the child's strengths and abilities; (3) soliciting the parental or guardian's view of the child's primary problems and needs; (4) history taking regarding the child's daily living and performance skills such as eating, sleeping, dressing, attention, etc.; (5) observing the child in his environment, and (6) administering standardized tests to explore or measure specific skills or abilities, or to discover underlying factors related to problem areas identified in parental interviews and observations.

Some of the most commonly used performance tests are listed in table 4.

Hypothesis Generation and Testing

The second stage in the occupational therapy process is to interpret the information gathered during the assessment phase. The stage consists of hypothesis generation and hypothesis testing. During hypothesis generation, the occupational therapist renders a hypothesis about how the child's unique configuration of functional and dysfunctional factors (skills and abilities) is affecting the occupational performance.

Table 2. Health problems of pediatric occupational therapy clients

Primary health problem	Patients, %
Cerebral palsy	31.7
Developmentally delayed	46.1
Adjustment disorder	2.1
Affective disorder	1.6
Mental retardation	8.5
Other[1]	10.0

[1] Amputation, burns, cancer, congenital abnormality, eating disorder, injuries, hearing disabled, spinal cord injury, visual disability, neonatal care, respiratory disorder, multiply handicapped, sensory integrative disorder.

Source: American Occupational Therapy Association, 1986, member survey [Unpubl. data]. Used with permission.

Table 3. Referral criteria for occupational therapy evaluation

Reason for referral	References
Delay in physical, cognitive, language or self help/self regulation ability	Hanft [6]
Poor nutritive/nonnutritive suck/swallow patterns of feeding or eating	Case-Smith et al. [7]
Excessive drooling, abnormal tongue use	Schwaab et al. [8]
Extreme or unusual reactions to non-noxious sensory experiences	Ayres [9]
Long-term hospitalization	Kielhofner et al. [10]
Need for device or equipment for eating postural control, hand use or mobility	Trefler et al. [11]
Presence of medical condition putting child at risk for physical, emotional or educational delay	Pratt and Allen [4]

Table 4. Common standardized tests used by occupational therapists

Age group years	Standardized test	Performance component(s) measured
2.75–5.7	Miller assessment for preschoolers [12]	overall assessment of cognitive, motor language, and sensory motor performance
3–5	DeGangi-Berke test of sensory integration [13]	postural mechanisms
4–8	Sensory integration and praxis tests [14]	praxis and sensory processing

Table 5. Overview of four theoretical references of pediatric occupational therapists [adapted from ref. 4]

Developmental	based upon the interaction between biological and psychological development and the environmental setting which promotes or inhibits the process of maturation
Neurodevelopmental	based upon the work of Carl and Bertha Bobath; a specialized modality of therapeutic handling is thought to facilitate desired movement patterns and postural control
Sensory Integrative	based upon the work of the late A. Jean Ayres, based upon a complex theory of how the brain organizes sensory information for use
Biomechanical	based on the principles of therapeutic exercise, the restoration and/or maintenance of joint range of motion, muscle strength, coordination and endurance

During assessment of a young mentally retarded child, for example, the occupational therapist may note how the environment influences the child's behavior. Determining that the child's attention to task decreases as environmental stimuli increase, the occupational therapist helps to determine how the environment can be modified to facilitate the acquisition of age-appropriate skills and abilities.

Hypothesis testing is simply exploring the child's reaction to a planned intervention to determine if the child's response confirms the hypothesis.

Intervention

The occupational therapy intervention plan in pediatric rehabilitation is commonly predicated on one or more of four theoretical models: developmental, neurodevelopmental, sensory integrative and biomechanical. Table 5 summarizes these theoretical models.

Evaluation of the Intervention

Success of occupational therapy intervention is based on change in the family function related to their handicapped child or change in skills and abilities of the child. Determination of change is accomplished through observation of the child in his environments, readministration of standardized tests (as appropriate), and interviews with parents and teachers. The occupational therapy program is either continued, revised or discontinued.

Discharge Planning

Discharge planning allows for a comfortable transition to greater independence by the child and family. Long-range follow-up is a component which allows any subsequent problems to be dealt with in a timely and efficient manner.

Intervention Strategies

The pediatric occupational therapist employs some combination of three types of services: (1) treatment of the child individually or in a group setting; (2) environmental adaptation to facilitate skills and abilities and/or to normalize the child's dysfunctions, and (3) change of the organizational system surrounding the child to mitigate effects of the dysfunctional skills and abilities, as well as to enhance the child's functional skills and abilities.

Treatment

Treatment may occur in a variety of settings (hospital, clinic, institution, or home) with varying frequency (usually 1–5 sessions per week). During treatment sessions, the therapist's goal is to increase the child's adaptive responses [1, 2] and to facilitate improved function and occupational performance. Thus, the occupational therapist may be working on improved eye-hand coordination skills in a child so that he or she can better fulfill the role of student. Or, the occupational therapist may work with the child on compensation strategies to mitigate the effects of a disability. In this case, the occupational therapist may be working with an upper extremities congenital amputee to develop skills in the use of the lower extremity for fine motor tasks and independence in feeding and dressing.

Other examples of treatment include: (1) sensory-motor play activities which tap vestibular, proprioceptive, visual and tactile systems to enhance neural system function and maturation. Such play reduces gravitational insecurity, promotes visual pursuits, improves emotional stability and improves the child's ability to execute tasks in an organized, sequential manner; (2) neuromuscular facilitation techniques prior to and during feeding activities to promote more normal suck/swallow patterns and to enhance weight gain in the developmentally delayed infant, and (3) training the older child with hemiplegia in the proper use of a night splint to prevent contracture and deformity.

Environmental Adaptation

Modifications to improve a child's functioning can be made in the environments in which the child lives, plays, and learns. Examples may include: (1) consultation with planners to modify playgrounds for disabled children [3]; (2) consultation with families to modify and adapt kitchens and bathrooms for children with wheelchairs, walkers or canes, and (3) consultation with nursing staff to reduce unnecessary stimuli in a high-risk nursery to allow high-risk and handicapped infants an opportunity to develop self-regulation for eating, sleeping and comforting.

Systems Change

The generalization of therapeutic principles and procedures into all aspects of the child's life is the goal of systems change. In pediatric occupational therapy, the targets of systems change most often are the family, the school setting, and the play environment. Examples of systems change intervention include: (1) helping the parents of a developmentally delayed preschool child understand realistic expectations and goals for the child; (2) identifying with a classroom teacher the best learning modalities for an elementary school child with cerebral palsy affecting motor performance and visual perception, and (3) guiding the parents of an infant with severe hypertonicity in using methods to handle their infant to influence better motor control during feeding, dressing and play.

Occupational Therapy Case Studies

Jenny

Jenny was a 3-year-old child diagnosed as having spastic quadriplegia. Increased muscle tone interfered with her ability to sit independently, be mobile, manipulate age-appropriate play materials, and use feeding utensils. She had normal intellectual and language development, but her speech was irregular due to abnormal muscle tone. She attended a mainstreamed pre-school program offering additional occupational, physical and speech therapy. Her home environment was responsive and supportive.

In the individual treatment, the occupational therapist employed neurodevelopmental techniques during specific play activities to improve Jenny's functional mobility, particularly in the execution of upper-extremity movements while Jenny was prone, sitting, and standing with support. Skill training in getting onto and off a potty seat, and the use of feeding utensils for increased independence was provided.

To apply therapeutic principles across settings (systems change), the occupational therapist coordinated with Jenny's classroom teacher to: (1) increase Jenny's independence at school, and (2) to increase her participation in school activities with other children. Various seating adaptations were devised to allow Jenny to sit independently in a variety of school settings. The occupational therapist constructed three specially designed seats for Jenny – one for floor activities, one for toileting, and one for tabletop activities and eating. Since drawing and painting were difficult for Jenny, a specifically adapted easel also was made for the use at school.

The occupational therapist further collaborated with the classroom teacher and guided the teacher in facilitation techniques to promote Jenny's independent functional mobility, eye-hand coordination, and self-care ability.

Although Jenny's family was supportive, her social interactions with peers were limited. The occupational therapist worked with the family to devise methods for assisting her in playing at the neighborhood playground on existing equipment.

Andrew

Andrew was born at 32-weeks gestational age, weighing 1,300 g. He suffered from mild respiratory distress syndrome and for 1 week received mechanical ventilation. The following was noted when Andrew was 6 months of age (4 months corrected age): low muscle tone, social and motor delay, poor nutritive sucking, and excessive irritability. Andrew's single, young mother lacked a high school education and received public assistance.

The mother's major concerns were Andrew's irritability and poor feeding. The therapist guided the mother to better understand how Andrew communicated distress and how to handle him using sensory integrative and neurodevelopmental techniques. The mother learned how to hold Andrew employing firm, predictable, and rhythmical rocking; Andrew would shift to a state of calm alertness when his mother held him in this manner. Improved mother-infant interaction set the stage for Andrew to improve feeding and bonding with his mother.

Andrew's poor oral motor and jaw control resulted in significant milk loss while feeding. The mother was frustrated because it took Andrew at least 45 min to eat. The occupational therapist tested the effectiveness of oral motor facilitation techniques with Andrew. He responded with improved feeding, and the therapist worked with the mother to carry on this oral motor facilitation at home.

The occupational therapist also directed treatment to improve Andrew's head control, eye tracking, and arm use. The mother learned from the occupational therapist how to play with Andrew in ways that facilitated the improvement in these deficit areas. Additionally, the occupational therapist helped to improve the mother's confidence in her ability to raise Andrew, a child with special needs.

Daniel

Five-year-old Daniel developed normally until the sudden onset of encephalitis. Referred to occupational therapy while still in a coma, he had random, uncontrolled movements with rigid muscle tone. He did not respond to visual, tactile or auditory stimuli. The initial goals of occupational therapy were the maintenance of joint and muscle integrity to prevent contractures and monitor sensory return.

The occupational therapist made lower-extremity splints and coordinated the care and use of the splints with the nursing staff. As Daniel began to acquire sensory and motor abilities, the occupational therapist monitored and facilitated his improvement. For example, the occupational therapist worked with Daniel in getting into and out of a chair. As oral motor control returned, the occupational therapist assisted Daniel in relearning how to eat and drink, progressing from finger to solid foods.

Summary

Occupational therapy in pediatric rehabilitation is directed to facilitate children's performance of self-care, work and leisure occupations in the context of daily life. The ultimate goal of occupational therapy is the development of the children's ability to function as independently as possible as they assume a variety of 'occupational' roles such as family member, student, and playmate.

Acknowledgement

Partial support for this project was made possible by the Pain Control Fund of the Department of Rehabilitation Medicine at The New York Hospital-Cornell Medical Center.

References

1 King, L.J.: Toward a science of adaptive response. Am. J. occup. Ther. *32:* 429–437 (1978).
2 Kleinman, B.L.; Bulkley, B.L.: Some implications of a science of adaptive responses. Am. J. occup. Ther. *36:* 15–19 (1982).
3 Stout, J.: Planning playgrounds for children. Am. J. occup. Ther. *42:* 653–657 (1988).
4 Pratt, P.N.; Allen, A.S.: Occupational therapy for children; 2nd ed (Mosby, St. Louis 1989).
5 Uniform Terminology (draft): Am. Occupational Therapy Ass., Rockville, 1989.
6 Hanft, B.H.: The clinician as advocate for sensory integration. Occup. Ther. Health Care *4:* 137–146 (1987).
7 Case-Smith, J.; Cooper, P.; Scala, V.: Feeding efficiency premature infants. Am. J. occup. Ther. *43:* 245–250 (1989).
8 Schwaab, M.; Niman, C.; Gisel, E.: Comparison of chewing cycles in 2-, 3-, and 5-year-old normal children. Am. J. occup. Ther. *40:* 40–43, (1986).
9 Ayres, A.J.: Sensory integration and the child (Western Psychological Services, Los Angeles 1979).
10 Kielhofner, G.; Barris, R.; Bauer, P.; Schoestock, B.; Walker, L.: A comparison of play behavior in nonhospitalized and hospitalized children. Am J. occup. Ther. *36:* 305–312, (1983).
11 Trefler, E.; Nickey, J.; Hobsen, D.: Technology in the education of multiple-handicapped children. Am. J. occup. Ther. *37:* 381–387 (1983).
12 Miller, L.J.: Miller assessment for preschoolers-manual; rev. ed. (Psychological Corporation, San Antonio 1988).
13 DeGangi, G.; Berke, R.: Test of sensory integration (Western Psychological Services, Los Angeles 1983).
14 Ayres, A.J.: Sensory integration and praxis tests. (Western Psychological Services, Los Angeles 1989).

Received: October 23, 1989

Charlotte Brasic Royeen, PhD
American Occupational Therapy Association
1383 Piccard Drive
Rockville, VA 20850 (USA)

Pediatrician 1990;17:283–286

0300–1245/90/0174–0283$2.75/0

The Changing Role of the Speech-Language Pathologist in Pediatric Rehabilitation/Habilitation

Judy Gardner[a], *Marilyn Seif Workinger*[b]

[a]DuPage Easter Seal, Villa Park, Ill.; [b]Marshfield Clinic, Marshfield, Wisc., USA

Key Words. Language disorders · Feeding problems · Speech and voice disorders

Abstract. The speech-language pathologist shares in the management of children who have a need for pediatric rehabilitation/habilitation services. Technological advances provide new tools to assess and promote communication.

Introduction

The role of the speech-language pathologist in pediatric rehabilitation/habilitation has changed with the advent of technological advancements for children with communication disorders. Speech-language pathologists are professionals who hold either the master's or doctoral degree and are qualified to identify, assess, and provide treatment for individuals with speech, language, and/or hearing disorders. As Steven C. White from the ASHA National Office said, 'Speech-language pathologists are specialists in the understanding and expression of human communication, its normal development, its disorders, and the prevention of its disorders.' The speech-language pathologist works most effectively as a member of a team in a rehabilitation setting.

Disorders

The four most common areas of remediation in pediatric rehabilitative settings are feeding problems, language disorders, speech and voice disorders, and stuttering disorders.

Feeding Disorders

Early intervention by speech-language pathologists is now a widely accepted practice in the treatment of feeding problems. Many children have feeding problems either from birth, or due to injury following birth. Some of the fine motor movements required for sucking, swallowing, biting, and chewing are also those needed for the production of speech sounds [1]. The goal of involving a child in a feeding program as early as possible (preferably before 1 year of age) is to prevent oral deformities and abnormal motor patterns and possibly prepare the child for more normal speech production. An example of feeding therapy would be with Andrew, an 11-month-old child with severe athetoid cerebral palsy. With correct positioning and inhibition of abnormal jaw- and tongue-thrusting patterns, Andrew is able to cup drink and chew table foods with movement patterns similar to those of a normal 11-month-old (fig. 1). By activating correct lip closure and tongue elevation at a normal motor developmental level, much of the drooling and abnormal oral motor movements of the child with cerebral palsy can be prevented.

The speech-language pathologist works with the child to inhibit abnormal feeding, respiratory, and phonatory patterns and to promote more normal oral motor activities. Using the modified barium swallow videofluoroscopic examination, the speech-language pathologist working with the radiologist can determine the extent and the nature of the feeding problem [2]. Baseline evaluations and comparison studies can be done to structure the treatment program. Children who aspirate or those at risk for aspiration can be identified to allow for early intervention. Structural anomalies also can be identified using the video fluoroscopic exam.

Language Disorders

Language can be defined as the method of communicating thought and feeling whether through gestures, facial expression or words. Children may have language disorders of input (hearing impairment, visual impairment), disorders of central nervous system processing (head trauma, mental retardation, developmental language disorders), or disorders of output (dysarthria, anatomic abnormalities of the vocal tract) [3, 4].

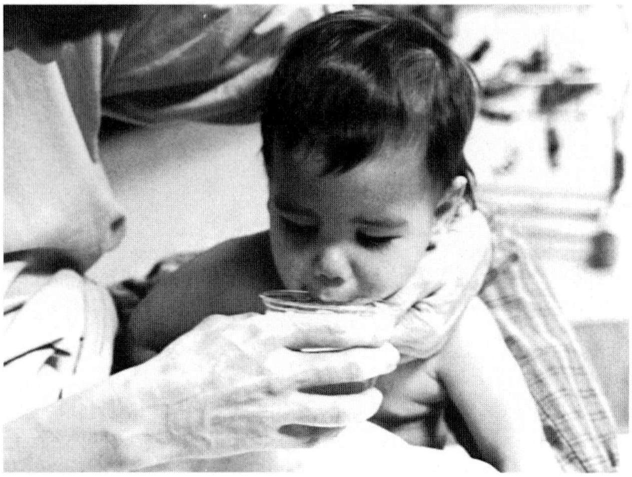

Fig. 1. Feeding therapy with an 11-month-old child with cerebral palsy to inhibit abnormal motor patterns.

Computers are having far-reaching effects in language therapy. Programs exist for problems as simple as cause-effect and as complex as sophisticated language. The complexity and sophistication of computer-driven devices with voice output is now available to children whose cognitive potential allows their use. Augmentative speech communication systems provide new opportunities for the severely speech-impaired and language-disordered population. These communication systems are most commonly used with the dysarthric cerebral-palsied child. Augmentative systems also have been used with language-delayed and language-deviant children, including those who are cognitively impaired and autistic [3]. One system (called 'Minspeak') allows the user to employ computerized speech via icons (pictorial representation of ideas), and allows the speaker to communicate in thoughts, not just word utterances [5]. Tina is an 11-year-old child with hearing impairment and cerebral palsy (dysarthric). Her speech is primarily unintelligible to an outside listener. Tina uses a 'Touch Talker' (fig. 2) with 'Minspeak' vocabulary. She has a vocabulary of 1,000 words and phrases with a voice synthesizer output. Tina is ambulatory but unable to carry her portable device. The Touch Talker is mounted on a wheeled cart

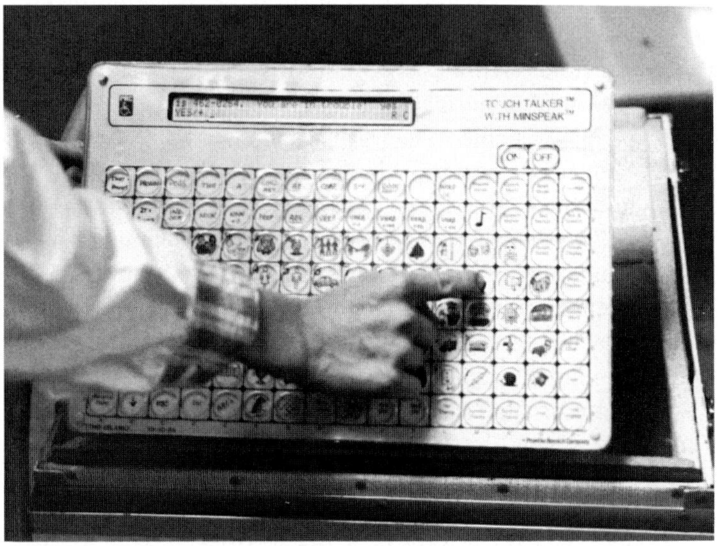

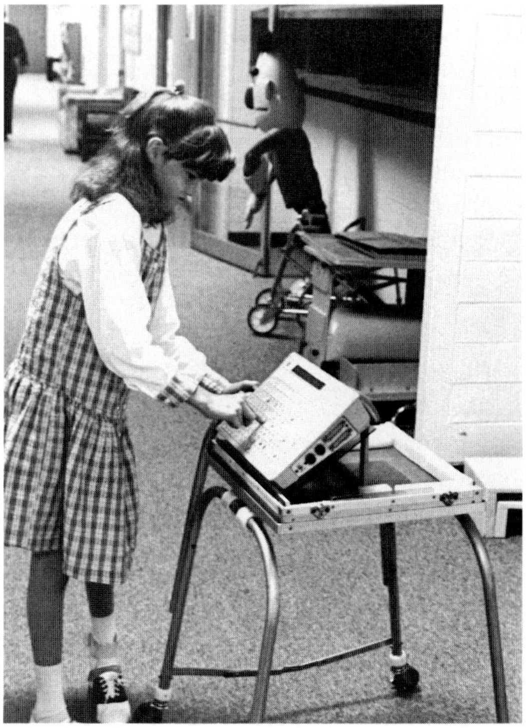

Fig. 2. Eleven-year-old child using a Touch Talker for augmentative communication.

to go from class to class. Tina is now totally mainstreamed into normal classes. She is also able to interface her Touch Talker to an Apple computer to generate hard copy for her homework. Computer models of the human mind are being developed with particular attention being placed on how those models might learn and communicate. The use of artificial intelligence will have far-reaching effects on the future of speech-language therapy for children with communication disorders. A program called 'Mindreader' (Telemarketing Resources, Campbell, Calif., USA) is a word processor that predicts the next word to be typed, corrects spelling, grammar, and recalls the style of composing for future reference.

Speech and Voice Disorders

The speech mechanism can be thought of as a series of components including the abdomen, diaphragm, larynx, velopharynx, tongue, jaw and lips. These components work individually or in combination to generate an air stream and to valve that air stream [6]. Air pressure and air flow can be measured during speech production to assess the integrity of the respiratory support system and the efficiency of valving at the larynx and velopharynx. The child who makes an error on the final sound in the word 'house' is showing an articulatory error. To evaluate the cause for this error and to develop an appropriate treatment program, the speech pathologist must be prepared to assess multiple speech subsystems in additon to making perceptual judgments. The child's speech error could be due to one or more causes; it could be developmental in nature, part of a phonological disorder, secondary to a structural anomaly or the result of a speech motor control disorder.

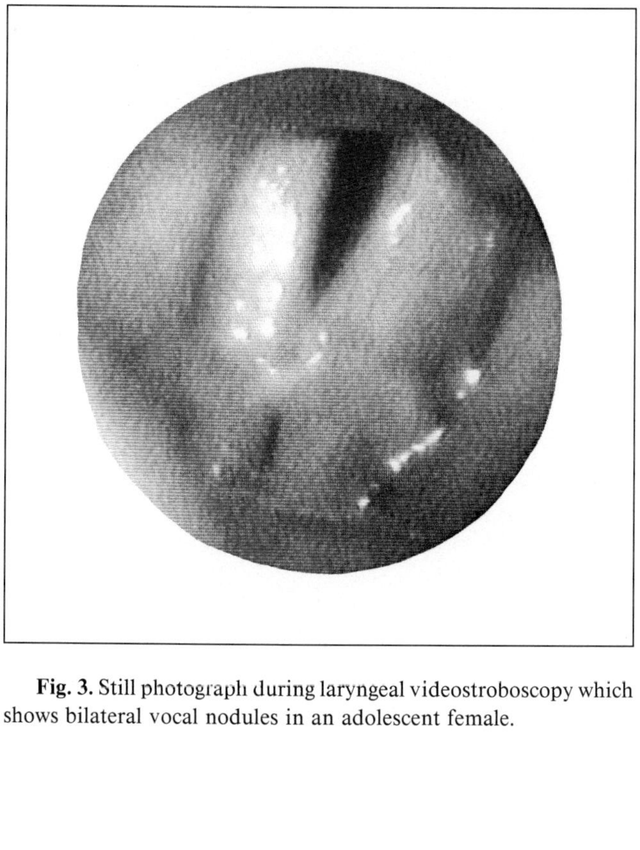

Fig. 3. Still photograph during laryngeal videostroboscopy which shows bilateral vocal nodules in an adolescent female.

Visual examination of the larynx during speech production can be accomplished through the use of techniques such as videostroboscopy (fig. 3). Vocal intensity, fundamental frequency and other parameters of pitch and nasality can all be quantified [7]. Nasendoscopy and videofluoroscopy allow the evaluation of velopharyngeal port functions during speech production [8]. Many of these tools can be used to assess the effect of medical intervention such as surgical procedures to repair clefts of the hard and soft palate. All the procedures described can be performed on children as young as 4 years of age.

Stuttering

Stuttering is a communication disorder characterized by excessive involuntary disruptions or blockings in the flow of speech, particularly when such disruptions consist of repetitions or prolongations of a sound or syllable, and when they are accompanied by avoidance struggle behavior. Technology has facilitated advances in the treatment of this speech disorder. Devices such as masking and delayed auditory feedback have been used to reduce the effect of the characteristics of stuttering. Computers are being used to provide a training for the shaping of precision fluency. The therapist uses a computer program to teach the stutterer a basic tutorial in controlling stuttering and auditory training skills, and then monitors the patient's voice onset. This computerized training program is having a 90% success rate with an intensive 19-day therapy program [9].

Summary

The role of the speech-language pathologist in rehabilitation/habilitation settings is changing with the evolution of new technology. Feeding disorders, language disorders, speech and voice disorders, and stuttering are four major areas of pediatric rehabilitation. Technology allows the speech-language pathologist a more sophisticated and objective evaluation of children with speech-language and feeding disorders, and a better documentation of progress or a lack of progress. Speech-language treatment at times involves alternative or augmentative communication systems, and the quantity and quality of devices available to the therapist is increasing rapidly.

References

1 Alexander RP: A cineflurographic investigation of jaw, lip and tongue movements in oral functions and speech in normal adults; unpublished thesis. University of Illinois, 1976.
2 Logemann J: Evaluation and Treatment of Swallowing Disorders. San Diego, College-Hill Press 1983.
3 Miller J, Yoder D, Schiefelbusch R, et al: Contemporary Issues in Language Intervention. Rockville, ASHA Reports 12, 1983.
4 Coplan J: Speech and language development. Pediatr Ann 1985; 14:3.
5 Baker B: Using images to generate speech. Byte 1986;3.
6 Netsell R: Speech physiology; in Minifie F, Hixon T, Wiliams F (eds): Normal Aspects of Speech, Hearing and Language. Englewood Cliffs, Prentice-Hall 1973.
7 Baken R: Clinical Measurement of Speech and Voice, San Diego, College-Hill Press 1987.
8 McWilliams B, Morris H, Shelton R: Cleft Palate Speech. Philadelphia, Decker 1984.
9 Webster R: Stuttering Then and Now. Columbus, Merrill 1986.

Received: December 1, 1989

Judy Gardner
Director of Communication Disorders
DuPage Easter Seal
Villa Park, IL 60181 (USA)

Pediatrician 1990;17:287–296

0300–1245/90/0174–0287$2.75/0

Rehabilitation Engineering in Pediatrics

M. Milner, S. Naumann, W. Literowich, M. Martin, S. Ryan, W.F. Sauter, G.F. Shein, G. Verburg

Rehabilitation Engineering Department, The Hugh MacMillan Rehabilitation Centre, Toronto, Ontario, Canada

Key Words. Communication aids · Computers · Mobility · Myoelectric prostheses · Orthotics · Prostheses · Postural support · Seating

Abstract. Applications of science and technology in the (re)habilitation of children and young adults can have dramatic, positive influences on their lives. Prosthetics, orthotics, mobility, postural support and seating, communication and education are responsibilities of the rehabilitation engineer. A holistic approach in meeting individual needs for technology is essential. The concerted rehabilitation engineering programme at The Hugh MacMillan Rehabilitation Centre supports service programmes with relevant research and development work.

Introduction

Wise applications of technology can have dramatic, positive effects on the lives of children with congenital or acquired disabilities, their families and communities [1]. Modern technology has facilitated functional capability through prosthetics and orthotics. Externally powered prostheses and orthoses have been developed; experimentation with artificial stimulation of muscle to yield functional capabilities is promising. Mobility often is enhanced by prosthetic or orthotic systems. Wheelchairs and specialized seating systems can promote independence in mobility and opportunities to access technology for powered mobility, education, vocation, recreation or leisure. Powered mobility might include automobiles with modifications to permit individuals independent transportation in the wider community.

Technology can, to some extent, compensate for sensory losses such as vision or hearing. Hearing and visual aids are relying more on microminiaturized electronic systems, and greater use is being made of computer-based technology. For non-speaking individuals and others with speech impediments, computer-based technology is contributing enormously to their opportunities and capabilities for communication.

Many children with disabilities will require life-long support from their families, the community and rehabilitation specialists. The complexity and subtlety involved in providing many technical aids demand a holistic approach in dealing with each individual's needs.

The environment and circumstances in which individuals function must be understood to direct efforts toward the goals of maximum independence and life satisfaction. Understanding the developmental phases in an individual's life, both physical and cognitive, is essential. Thus, the provision of effective rehabilitation technology is not the preserve of engineers and technologists alone. Many other disciplines – physicians, physical and occupational therapists, psychologists, nurses, vocational counsellors, educators – contribute significantly.

In many countries, specialists in rehabilitation engineering are emerging through experience with particular clinical programmes, but in rarer instances with formal educational training. Rehabilitation engineering is con-

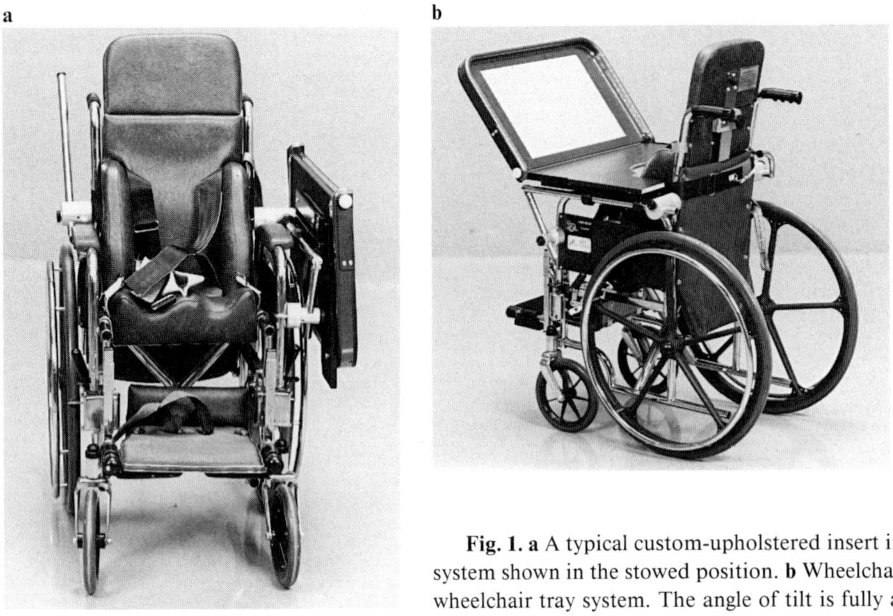

Fig. 1. a A typical custom-upholstered insert in a wheelchair with a newly developed tray system shown in the stowed position. b Wheelchair fitted with insert and tiltable swing-away wheelchair tray system. The angle of tilt is fully adjustable from horizontal to upright.

cerned with the infusion of appropriate levels of science and technology in the (re)habilitative process.

At The Hugh MacMillan Rehabilitation Centre (HMRC) in Toronto, a concerted rehabilitation engineering programme for youngsters with physical disabilities provides patient service programmes relating to postural support and seating, mobility and special controls, augmentative communications, prosthetics, orthotics and educational needs. Efforts are continually made to underpin each service or programme with relevant research and development work to ensure efficiency of operations and the effective utilization of the most modern technology.

Postural Support and Seating Systems

These systems can be considered to be the underpinnings of most rehabilitation programmes in which the individual requires an insert in a wheeled base for mobility or for other needs relating to personal transportation. Neuromusculoskeletal deficiencies can, to some degree, be countered by effective, well-designed systems. Positioning for the management of orthopaedic deformities is of crucial importance. Other goals include cosmesis, opportunities to effectively control (powered) mobility and communication systems including environmental controllers, opportunities for self-feeding, play and education. Pressure-diffusing cushion surfaces play an important role in tissue trauma management. Specialized trays affixed to wheelchairs can provide upper body support, can serve as a feeding table, a support for reading or writing materials, or a pictographic communication board. Technical aids including portable computers, voice synthesisers or controllers for commanding externally powered mobility can be supported by or fixed to the tray.

Service Programme

The interaction between services which work towards provision of devices in each of these areas requires concert and special attention for efficient address of the child's needs. Avoidance of fragmentation of such services and assurance of geographic proximity are important. The orthopaedic surgeon, occupational therapist, rehabilitation technologist and consultant rehabilitation engineer integrate the overall needs of the individual to generate a seating design. If other services are likely to impact on the design, their inputs are sought. The design is passed on to the workshop where most of the custom work is in wood and foams including polystyrene liquid foam for intimate contouring. Expert custom upholsterers assure an aesthetic quality product. Other commercially available systems such as Canadian Posture and Seating, Otto Bock and Special Health Systems are prescribed and fabricated as appropriate. Although at times requiring extensive custom work, parts of each system can be combined to meet specific needs of clients. Final upholstery covering of each seating system, usually with Naugahyde, follows

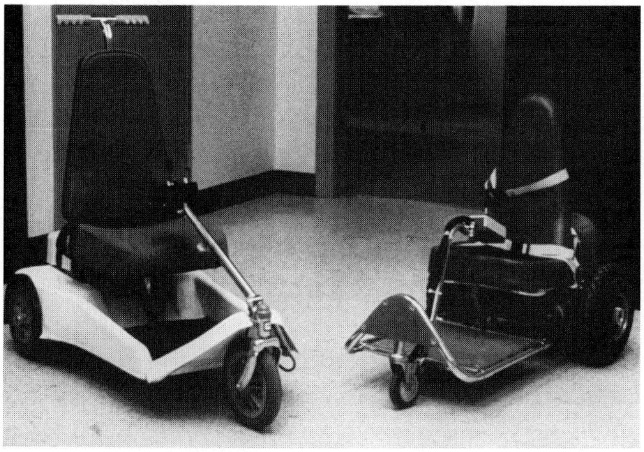

a

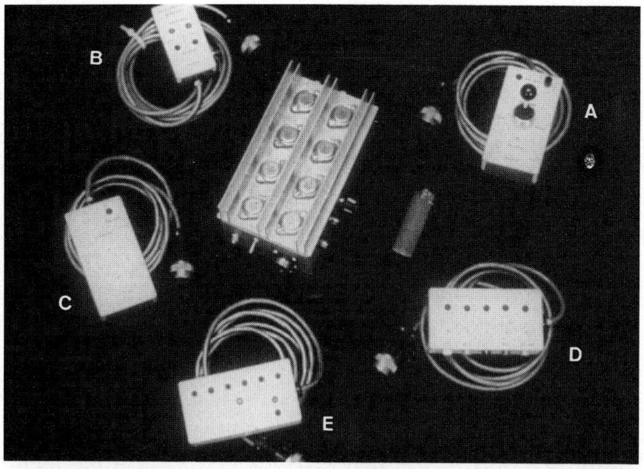

b

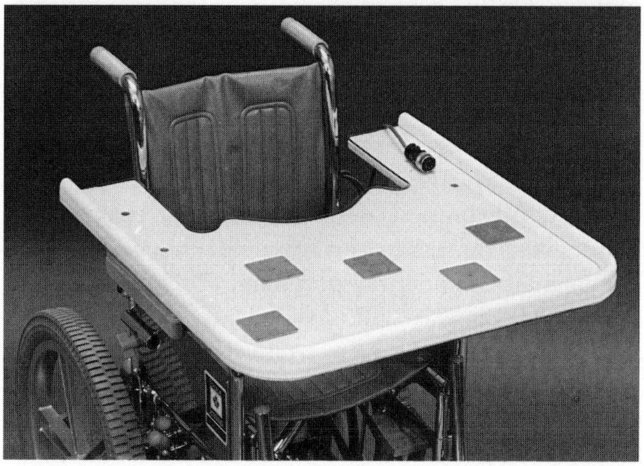

c

Fig. 2. **a** Prototype miniature-powered vehicle developed at HMRC (right) and Everest and Jennings production model (left). **b** Control systems. A = Regular joystick; B = head position control, using an arrangement of mercury switches which can be attached to the head. Head movements provide directional commands to a powered wheelchair; C = a touch-plate system for individuals with limited digit movements allows for selection of directional commands; D = another touch-plate system allows for flexible placement of touch-plates to permit control by individuals with large-range athetoid movements (fig. 2c); E = a scanning selector system programmed to illuminate sequentially the directional commands forward, backward, left and right through the action of a single switch. Individuals with very severe physical limitations can use this. **c** Touch-plates on a tray to command wheelchair directions by individuals with large-range athetoid movements.

after trial periods to assure that the individual's seating goals are met.

Quality assurance procedures facilitate the informed use and safety of the devices. Each completed product is inspected for quality of workmanship, adherence to the original prescription and safety standards. Written and/or verbal instructions are provided to caregivers and clients in the use and maintenance of the device. Figure 1a shows a typical custom-upholstered insert.

In 1988, over 550 children and young adults were assessed, 355 new systems were prescribed, and 345 inserts, trays and bases were modified for growth and/or changes in medical or environmental need.

Research and Development at HMRC

Recent developments include a Kydex tiltable swing-away wheelchair tray system [2] (fig. 1), a universal joystick/tray mount, tiltable armrest brackets, and a tiltable seating interface to fit most current wheelchair models while still allowing it to fold.

Current research includes addressing issues relating to anteriorly tipped seating for mild to moderately involved children with cerebral palsy, the use of saddle type seats, and the development of additional modular seating components to help reduce costs.

Personalized Transportation and Mobility Systems

Of importance in prescribing powered wheelchairs is an understanding of the circumstances and environments in which the individual will use the device. Knowledge of specific community needs, schooling, and the domestic environment is necessary. Individuals who lack upper extremity strength and control of movements often will require powered wheelchairs. Units emerging are capable of negotiating rough terrain and perhaps even stairs. The provision of control systems other than regular joysticks has widened the possibilities of mobility particularly for severely disabled persons (fig. 2). Systems now are available with scanning options for directional controls selected by activating a single switch. Switching arrangements can assist individuals with limited ranges of movement as well as large flailing movements.

Children with severe physical disabilities precluding the possibility for hand-propelled mobility can use battery-powered mobility aids with appropriate control systems (fig. 2). Children as young as 2 years of age have used these devices responsibly, and have become more outgoing, exploratory, and thus more favourably competitive with their peers.

Computer-based assessments and training of skill for mobility control are being developed. Training techniques are being devised to minimize the time for mastering of safe, efficient wheelchair control. The incorporation of 'intelligent' control systems to minimize the control burden on severely physically disabled persons (e.g. systems to assure steering along a straight line once a particular direction of travel has been selected) is being explored. Customized controls for steering, braking, signalling, and transmission can provide independence in personal automobile transportation. For wheelchair users requiring special lifting systems for access to their vehicles, tie-down systems ensure the stability of their wheelchairs while in place behind the driver's wheel or its equivalent. Again, provision of appropriate assessment services, technological design and individual training are the ingredients of a successful outcome.

Service Programme at HMRC

Forty to fifty new customized systems, touch trays for large flailing athetoid movements and touch-plate systems for those with limited ranges of movements of digits (fig. 2) have been created. Support is provided also for a specialised programme of Driver Education so that individuals with congenital or acquired disabilities can have independence in the use of automobiles.

Research and Development

Computer-based technological devices and mobility aids are providing new opportunities for the handicapped. Voice recognition systems to aid individuals with quadriplegia have been developed which enable environmental control and operation and programming of computers to be achieved. A scanning system for use in automobiles by high-level quadriplegics to control auxillary functions (e.g. wipers, signals, horn and lighting operations) is being refined and should be commercially available in the future [3].

Cognitive and physical issues are of importance in meeting the needs of children and young adults. Cognitive development includes motor, perceptual and symbolic learning and development. Learning and developmental needs of the young often are underestimated.

To facilitate their learning experiences, children with spina bifida, at the earliest possible stages, have been placed in caster carts (micro-wheelchairs) which they can propel independently. The benefits have been substantial for children with upper extremity limitations as well. In cases of spinal muscular atrophy and cerebral palsy, miniature-powered vehicles have great value. This was observed in a study in which ten 2- to 5-year-old children each were given a minature-powered vehicle for use at home and/or school. In the 1 year during which these children were followed they made statistically significant gains in social and academic skills and showed improvements in communication skills [4].

In a recent mobility-related project [5] physically and cognitively impaired students were given trainer units to take home. These units are interactive and the training programme can be modified via a modem link between HMRC and the student's home. Sixteen subjects have been provided with trainer units. Four of the 16 already have reached the level of training with 4 switches. At least 1 of the subjects has shown significant gain in the periodic wheelchair assessments. Participating children, parents and teachers have indicated excitement with the project.

Augmentative and Alternative Communication via Computer-Based Technology

Aids to support non-speaking, physically disabled individuals are of major importance. The emergence of microcomputer-based systems for communication and control purposes is having dramatic effects on the lives of these people by providing a communication capability and means of expression in language conveyed by speech synthesizers and through the creation of drawings and sketches, and the generation of music. Figure 3 shows computer-generated artwork created by a severely physically disabled non-speaking youngster. The user must control only one variable, that is whether a switch is on or off, to communicate with and to control a computer.

For a computer to present options to the individual for selection, a switch operated at the right moment can have enormous empowering consequences. A wide variety of input devices designed to overcome the disadvantages of different kinds and levels of disability is available. There are single or multiple switches, joysticks, hand- and head-pointing devices, touch tablets, expanded and miniature keyboards, voice and eyegaze control systems. The challenges faced in design and development relate to the assurance of access to computer-based devices for individuals with disabilities, the need to speed up the interactive communication process, and the enhancement of assessment and prescriptive capabilities.

Computer systems can contribute substantially to environmental control. The widespread use of computer systems for non-disabled persons enhances the opportunities for economic exploitation of such systems to benefit persons with disabilities. Advocacy for the needs of disabled persons must be sustained to avoid limitations that might be presented by developers of technology who lack experience with special populations.

Computerized aids augment the work of speech pathologists by providing exciting challenges and rewards for success through carefully contrived graphical displays. By providing visual feedback to speech-impaired children under the control of the speech pathologist, there is significant potential for strengthening individual rehabilitative programmes while expanding the capabilities of the speech pathologist.

The incorporation of voice synthesis in computer systems has had an impact upon persons with blindness and visual impairments.

Service Programme at HMRC

The Augmentative Communication Service (ACS) targets children who are non-speaking. Consultative, educational, prescriptive and training expertise is provided through a service delivery model which relies heavily on committed support of external facilitators who are usually significant in the child's life. Rehabilitation engineering and scientific engineering developmental support is provided to this programme. ACS provides a considerable amount of 'high-tech' expertise to scores of patients/clients, serviced annually with devices including computers and voice synthesizers.

Research and Development

The Microcomputer Applications Programme at HMRC embraces a multidisciplinary team supported by both ACS and the Rehabilitation Engineering Department. Efforts over the past 7 years have concentrated on developing systems to enable user access to computers and procedures for systematic clinical assessment of the individual user. The programme emphasises the need to meet varying needs of users recognising that there is no single 'best' configuration for an access system. Flexible access allowing users to realize their greatest potential is the goal.

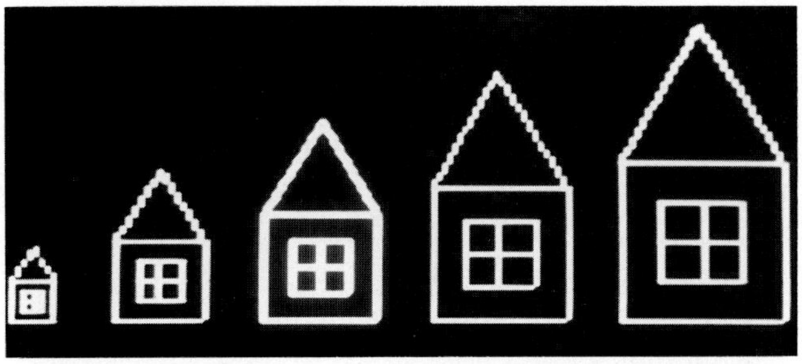

Fig. 3. Artwork generated by a youngster who had never held a pencil or crayon, using a computer controlled by a single switch.

A collaborative Shared Universities Research Project between the University of Toronto, HMRC, and International Business Machines Corporation has recently been completed (1985–1988). In this project, strategies were formulated for use by computer manufacturers and developers of alternate or non-standard access systems to ensure that people with wide-ranging disabilities could gain access to computers. The strategies consolidate clinical and technical knowledge gained through the clinicians' experience working with people with disabilities and computer technology. Strategies relate to issues of input, output, selection techniques, setup and configuration, and connecting to target computer systems. To demonstrate the application of these strategies, a model for an ideal alternate access system was designed and a clinical resource manual was created to help clinicians choose appropriate access systems for their clients. Present research relates to overcoming problems created by direct manipulation access systems; i.e., those requiring pointing devices such as a mouse.

Assessment

One issue that emerges when using computer technology is the need to appropriately assess people for their skills. A clinical resource manual specifically addresses this need [6]. It provides a systematic assessment process to assist clinicians in making well-informed decisions regarding the prescription, personalization and follow-up of access systems for their clients to achieve a 'best' possible control of computer-based technology. The assessment addresses the needs of people with primary motor disabilities such as cerebral palsy, spinal cord injury, amyotrophic lateral sclerosis, and muscular dystrophy. Sensory and cognitive impairments affect the assessment only when they co-occur with motor disabilities.

Expanded Vocabulary Augmentative Communication Device

The Expanded Vocabulary Augmentative Communication Device is a multifaceted communication aid designed and developed at HMRC for use by severely physically disabled non-speaking users. The device shown in figure 4 increases vocabulary display space by incorporating 9 removable prisms that provide approximately 540 square spaces for letters of the alphabet, words, pictures, and symbols. When the user depresses the externally mounted switch, the prism set is rotated 120 degrees to display 1 of 3 different surfaces. This device can be used on a tabletop, or a wheelchair tray, and is activated by a single switch. It is available as a product from Variety Ability Systems, Inc.

Prosthetics and Orthotics

Developments in these areas continue to advance with improvement in technology and exploitation of newer materials. Lightweight, electrically powered prosthetic hands and elbows (either myoelectrically or switch-controlled) are on the market and improvements in function continue to be developed. In the past decade, the trend has been to provide myoelectric fittings at earlier ages. In Toronto, children as young as 15 months have been fitted with below-elbow myoelectric prostheses. Close attention needs to be paid to the youngest users of all these systems to assess their full impact, particularly in functional terms, in later life. Computer systems are being used to facilitate the best electrode placement for myoelectrically controlled systems and for training and assessment purposes. The transfer of such technology into routine clinical practice requires specialized technical resources and well trained staff. Toronto experience indicates that if prosthetists do not specialize in this area, the likelihood of success with their fittings is considerably diminished.

Braces to promote functional capability are being enhanced by imaginative designers. Dynamic bracing and enhanced functional capability have evolved with developments in functional electrical stimulation of muscle. Muscles for which nervous control has been disrupted can be artificially stimulated to yield function.

Children with cerebral palsy undergoing corrective surgery to the lower extremities need to have orthotics fabricated and fitted almost immediately after such surgery. Long delays encountered in waiting for custom-made devices tend to mitigate against the value of the surgery. There is thus an indication for appropriate modular orthoses which can be readily and quickly fitted.

Service Programme at HMRC

The Powered Upper Extremity Prosthetics Programme (PUEPP) within the Rehabilitation Engineering Department and a separate Prosthetics/Orthotics De-

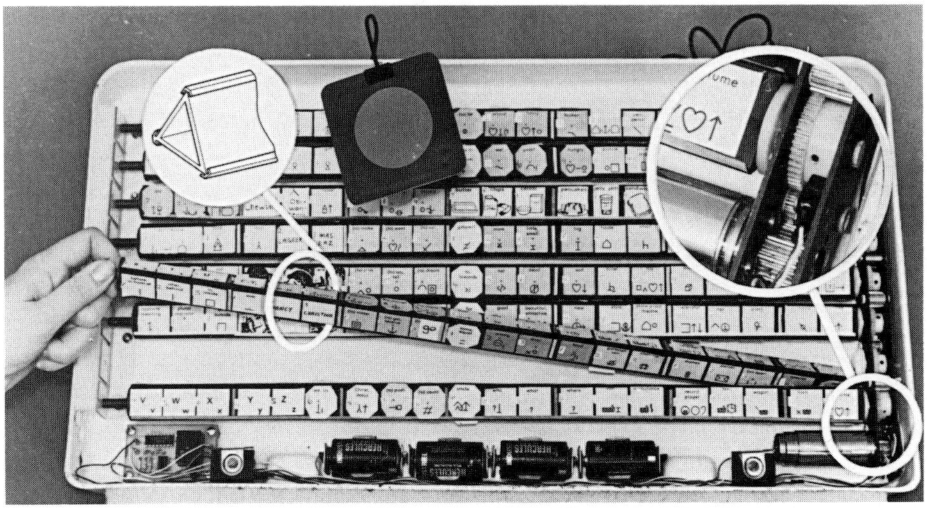

Fig. 4. Expanded Vocabulary Augmentative (EVA) Communication Device. This device can fit into the tray system shown in figure 1.

partment are responsible primarily for conventional upper extremity prosthetic fittings, lower extremity prostheses and orthoses of a wide variety. A multidisciplinary Amputee Programme embraces the strengths of orthopaedic and physiatry specialists, occupational therapists, a social worker and the various prosthetic services along with relevant developmental engineering support.

PUEPP's mandate is to provide consultation, design and development of relevant prosthetic components, control systems, and overall prostheses, and to fabricate and fit up-to-date electrically powered prostheses to children and young adults. The aim, consistent with all rehabilitation efforts, is to help each patient to achieve his or her maximum level of functional rehabilitation and integration into society. The programme has provided more than 1,300 electrically powered artificial arms to children and adults. These arms may be switch-controlled, myoelectrically controlled or hybrid systems, and are fitted to individuals with amputations ranging from single below-elbow to bilateral shoulder disarticulations. Linked intimately with the programme is a facility managed by the Rehabilitation Engineering Department called Variety Ability Systems Inc. (VASI) which manufactures and markets the products developed by PUEPP and the department.

Much of the success of this programme can be attributed to a teamwork approach, but the specially developed prosthetic fitting skills provide the essential technical means for sustaining a comfortable and functional fit of the prosthesis. Functional assessment and training aspects are largely the domain of the occupational therapist.

Research and Development

Technology transferred to VASI for manufacture and worldwide distribution includes the following electric hands and elbows (fig. 5).

VV0-3 Electric Hand. Designed for children aged 15–36 months and utilizing a plastic hand body and fingers to reduce the weight to 130 g, the hand provides the child

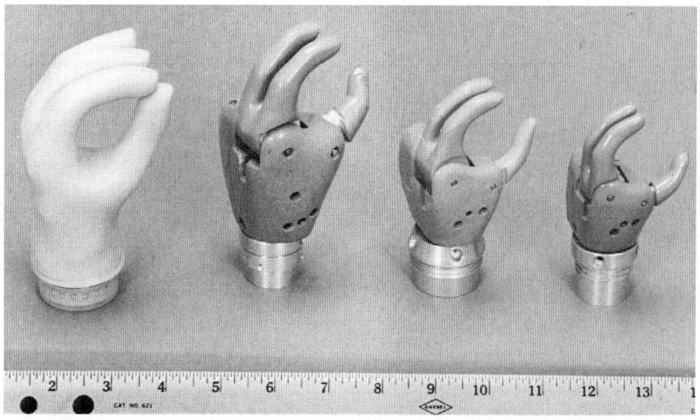

a

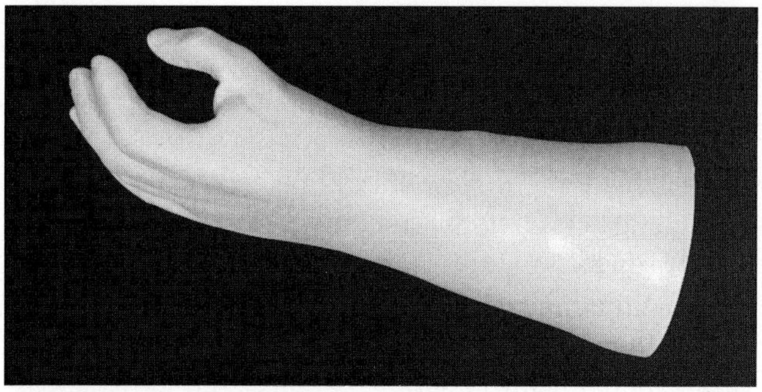
b

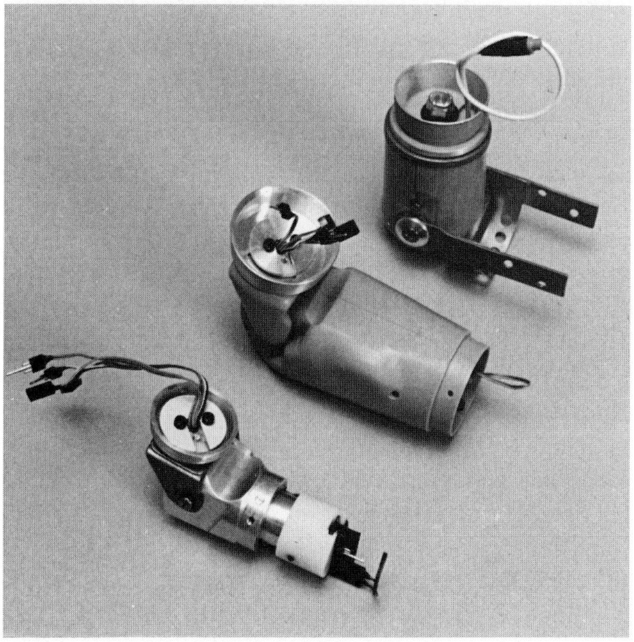
c

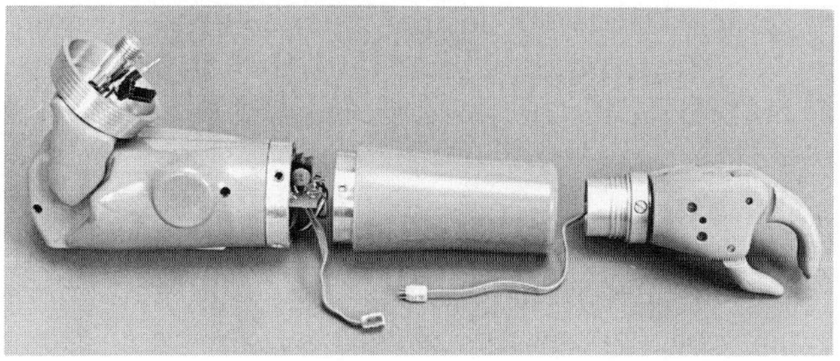
d

Fig. 5. a From right to left: VV0-3, VV2-6, VV5-9 and Otto Bock electric hands. All hands have a three-point pinch and are shown without cosmetic covers. **b** Latex rubber cosmetic cover for VV2-6 hand. **c** From left to right: VV3-8, VV8-12 and VV62 electric elbows. **d** Electric arm system with VV8-12 elbow, adjustable (by cutting to size) forearm and VV2-6 hand.

with the initial introduction to an electrically powered terminal device. More than 120 children worldwide are now using this device.

VV2-6 Electric Hand. As the first electric hand marketed by VASI in the current series since 1984, this has become popular in Canada and elsewhere. With over 275 hands now in service, this mid-size plastic hand weighing 168 g is continuing to give users reliable service.

VV5-9 Electric Hand. This hand, generally suited for children aged 5–9 years, completes the range of three lightweight hands to serve the needs of children from 15 months to approximately 10 years of age. Again lightweight because of the plastic components, it is similar in appearance and function to the VV2-6 version but 20% larger. It was introduced to the market in late 1989.

VV3-8 Electric Elbow. This minielbow, expected to be suitable for children as young as 2 years of age, is now being used by approximately 10 clients. Powered from a 6 volt source, and incorporating a partially prefabricated plastic forearm, this tiny device is expected to become very popular with children, parents, and prosthetists. The introduction of the minielbow will complete the range of elbows for children from the age of 2 through to the late teenage years.

VV8-12 Electric Elbow. With more than 25 of these electric elbows now in service, they have become very popular with children in the 7- to 12-year-old range. Again, a partially prefabricated forearm component is provided which allows for quick adjustment (shortening by cutting to size) and the fitting of a terminal device, and also provides space for the insertion of electronic systems for either switch- or myoelectric-control. This elbow incorporates a swing-free feature when in full extension.

VV62 Electric Elbow. This device for teenagers and adults has been available for many years and is available for 6 and 12 volt systems.

A recent project at HMRC [7] used microcomputers to establish objective standards and develop new strategies for the analysis of myoprosthetic operation. The project goals were: (1) to develop and test the reliability of an objective test of an amputee's ability to control a myoelectric control system; (2) to establish and develop a standard database of an amputee's ability to operate a myoelectric prosthesis; (3) to increase the speed and accuracy of the muscle site location and control system calibration procedures through the development of a microcomputer-based muscle-site identifier and control system calibrator; and (4) to evaluate the new myoelectric muscle-site identifier and control system calibrator against traditional methods.

The project is nearing completion with positive results in virtually all areas. The demographic database will provide an ongoing database structure for the collection of patient information arising from further clinic encounters.

Mechanical Design and Services

The Mechanical Design and Services Programme at HMRC provides coordinated design and fabrication services to clients of the Centre and participates in clinically oriented research and development projects [8]. Specialized mechanical services are available directly to Centre clients or indirectly through other departmental programmes.

Typically, members of the programme are called upon to attend a service clinic to consult with clinicians or need originators and suggest possible technical solutions for problems facing a specific client. Cost estimates of needed devices or modifications are provided. Following approval, the work proceeds. If necessary, informal in-house trials are conducted, alterations to the device are made, and the device is released for use. Feedback from users and caregivers is encouraged as experience is gained with the dispensed device. As an example of this process, a physical therapist from the Centre's Age 0–6 Therapy Unit met with programme members to discuss the walking needs of an 18-month-old girl with bilateral phocomelia of the upper extremities. The young girl had bilateral knee and ankle foot orthoses (KAFOs) with a pelvic band and was motivated to walk, but she lacked the stability and balance to do so unassisted. Commercially available walkers were unsuitable because of her size and limb shaping. This consultation led to the development of a growth-adjustable miniature horseshoe walker with a security strap across her back and a strap across each KAFO. Following an initial functional trial, minor adjustments were made and the device was dispensed. At the age of 4, she is now an independent walker in part due to the training and security she received while using her specialized walker.

Programme members also are presented with requirements for meeting the needs of more than one individual. Initial formulation of the general specifications is usually limited to a small core group of designers and the need originators. Development proceeds only if the conceptual design appears feasible in terms of function and recovery of development costs from the sale of additional units. Feedback from either structured or informal field trials serves as the basis for making design refinements. To illustrate this, staff from the HMRC School met with members of the Rehabilitation Engineering Department to discuss the need for fully accessible workstation furniture to accommodate both the educational and therapeutic needs of the student with a physical disability in the classroom. A detailed survey discovered that commercially available computer tables generally do not facilitate access nor do they promote proper positioning of the student with a physical disability. In response to this, a multidisciplinary team undertook the first phase of a project to develop fully accessible computer workstation furniture [9]. Its performance was evaluated and favorably received in several classroom settings. Negotiations with local vendors were undertaken to manufacture the furniture in quantity.

Often, clinical and technical staff identify significant areas of needed improvements in service delivery practices. If a review of existing and alternative approaches indicates that there is a need to develop a new system, then funding is sought from external sources. Devices developed through this process are usually intended to meet the needs of many disabled individuals in the order of 50 or more per annum. Once funding has been secured, detailed drawings are prepared and one or more prototypes are fabricated. The development is assessed usually through structured field testing when comments from the caregiver and clinician are solicited in a formalized way. Technical performance of the system is also documented. As an example of this, the Centre's Dental and Prosthetics/Orthotics Departments identified the need to develop a helmet which could provide children prone to falls with the same level of protection as custom-moulded helmets at significantly less expense. Sport helmets do not offer a suitable alternative, because these children require a different degree of protection. With initial support from the Hospital for Sick Children Foundation, an industrially fabricated helmet was developed [10]. The helmet, which consisted of three parts, permitted the orthotist to achieve a custom fit by adjusting the relative positions of the pieces and fastening them in place. The performance of the helmet was assessed with the assistance of 10 individuals who each wore one for 2 months. The evaluation demonstrated that the device was well received and with some modifications could be dispensed economically through the Prosthetics/Orthotics Department as well as at other Centres. Further funding has since been received through the National Health Research and Development Programme of Health and Welfare Canada to refine the design and develop additional sizes.

Discussion

Concert of Services

For effective rehabilitation engineering services, the overall technological needs of a child should be assessed together with a relevant clinical team (or teams) including the parents and caregivers relating directly to the child. Solutions are often costly and need to be evaluated on a trial and error basis even if the clinical team has considerable experience in service delivery. Technological systems should be age-appropriate, provision should be made for training to use devices and considerations regarding growth, subsequent adaptation and cost are of importance.

A facilitator who is in continual contact with the home environment, school or workplace and who will assume responsibility for 'trouble-shooting' systems in the field can be most helpful. This facilitator must be trained to provide both electrical and mechanical maintenance of the prescribed device. Reliability and rapid turnaround of maintenance services are essential. At the same time costs should be kept to a minimum. Often, disabled persons require funding from third party payers who are also concerned about cost-benefits. Those reponsible for providing rehabilitative services, and particularly technology, have a responsibility to attend to relevant documentation.

The most effective service delivery programmes are usually underpinned by pertinent research and development activities. Well-established clinical services should encourage meaningful testing of new devices or technological concepts in client management. Such capability can be of immense value for technology transfer to industry. Rehabilitation is a worldwide issue and rehabilitative devices can enjoy world markets.

Community Rehabilitation

Many individuals requiring rehabilitation engineering products and services are not sick and they need to be living independently in the community. Most rehabilitation programmes and related rehabilitation engineering are conducted in and through institutions, possibly ignoring the 'community' needs of the individual. Outreach programmes are likely to be of great importance in the future, providing individuals with services in their own communities.

Conclusion

Science and technology have significant present and future roles to play in providing technical solutions to the problems of (re)habilitation faced by our children. A number of areas demand our focused attention to aid children with physical disabilities in the future.

References

1 Milner, M.: Critical and emerging issues in rehabilitation engineering. Proc. 8th Annu. Int. Electric and Electronic Engineers, Engineering in med. Biol. Soc., pp. 30–32 (Fort Worth 1986).

2 Blackstein-Adler, S.; Ryan, S.; Parnes, P.; Naumann, S.: Towards further development of a modular wheelchair tray system for the severely physically disabled: Final report to National Health Research and Development Program, Health and Welfare Canada (1989).

3 Snell, E.; Shire, B.; Young, M.; Naumann, S.: A multifunction vehicular interface unit for quadriplegic drivers. Proc. ICAART 88, Int. Conf. Assoc. Rehab. Technology, pp. 36–37 (Montreal, Quebec 1988).

4 Verburg, G.; Snell, E.; Pilkington, M.; Milner, M.: Effects of powered mobility on young handicapped children and their families. Proc. 2nd Int. Conf. Rehab. Engineering, pp. 172–173 (Ottawa 1984).

5 Jarvis, S.; Naumann, S.; Verburg, G.: Mobility training research project. Interim reports to Ontario Mental Health Foundation (Toronto, Ontario 1989).

6 Lee, K.; Thomas, D.J.: Control of computer-based technology for people with physical disabilities: an assessment manual (University of Toronto Press, Toronto 1990).

7 Mifsud, M.; Hubbard, S.; Verburg, G.; Naumann, S.; Galway, H.R.; Milner, M.: Microcomputer-based myoelectric assessment system: Association of children's prosthetic-orthotic clinics (Abstract; in press).

8 Ryan, S.; Al-Temen, I.; Naumann, S.: Multilevel project strategies for the development of rehabilitation devices for the physically disabled. Proc. ICAART 88, Int. Conf. Assoc. Adv. Rehab. Technology, pp. 10–11 (1988).

9 Ryan, S.; Bowles, J.; Skidmore, S.; Verburg, G.: Toward the development of an accessible computer workstation and school desk for use in the classroom: assessment of the basic unit. Final report to Ministry of Education (Ontario 1988).

10 Hill, S.; Moran, R.; Bochmann, D.; Milner, M.; Singleton, D.; Belbin, T.; Giavedoni, B.: Development of a protective helmet for disabled people. Proc. 10th Annu. Conf. Rehab. Technology, pp. 213–215 (1987).

Received: November 2, 1989

Dr. M. Milner
The Hugh MacMillan Rehabilitation Centre
350 Rumsey Road
Toronto, Ontario M4G 1R8 (Canada)

Pediatrician 1990;17:297–307

0300–1245/90/0174–0297$2.75/0

Creating Therapeutic Camp and Recreation Programs for Children with Chronic Illness and Disabilities

Carol J. Page[a], *Joanne Pearson*[b]

[a] Handicapped Sports Program, Department of Physical Therapy;
[b] Oncology Wilderness Experience, Departments of Oncology and Nursing, The Children's Hospital, Denver, Colo., USA

Key Words. Camping · Children · Chronic illness · Disability · Program planning · Recreation · Sports

Abstract. Challenging 'out of hospital' participation in camping and recreational activities has a significant impact on the lives of children with chronic illness and disabilities. Planning these special programs requires attention to resources, population needs, staff training, financing, equipment needs, liability issues and participant selection.

History of Sports for the Handicapped

World War II played a significant role in the development of recreation programs for handicapped European war veterans. Amputee ski programs in Europe and the Stoke Mandeville Wheelchair Games in England were among the first special programs. US war veterans initiated similar programs in America. As a result, the Paralyzed Veteran's Association and the National Handicapped Sports Association have been instrumental in promoting programs for disabled individuals in the US. The Cheff Center in Augusta, Mich., is a leader today in horseback riding for the handicapped. A world-renown innovative ski program is the National Sports Center for the Disabled at Winter Park Resort, Winter Park, Colo., USA. Leadership in therapeutic wilderness experiences is also found in Colorado at the Breckenridge Outdoor Education Center (BOEC).

In this paper, we will present profiles of two resources developed to meet the needs of disabled individuals, discuss the philosophy and program planning required to establish special needs programs, and provide several examples of specialized camps and programs.

Resource Profiles

The BOEC responds to the needs of physically disabled and chronically ill people through therapeutic wilderness experiences. The BOEC programs aim to empower these individuals to have more control over their lives, and therefore to play a more significant role in society.

BOEC was established in 1976 following the concept of Ski for Light for the blind and the Bitzolen Sports Program in Norway which developed ski and sports programs for disabled people. These programs provided the impetus for the BOEC's developing a therapeutic wilderness experience using the natural elements of the wilderness and outdoor adventure activities.

The strength of BOEC relates directly to the staff and interns who undergo extensive training to understand the needs of various special needs populations. This training enables the staff to develop individualized programs to effect client change. The core of the program emphasizes group support, living in a community, and individualized counselling. These tools, combined with challenging outdoor activities, build confidence and self-esteem as well as independence and autonomy. Individuals with physical disabilities are faced with issues influencing self-esteem, independence and productivity. BOEC employs adaptive ski experiences (including monoskiing and sit skiing) and therapeutic wilderness programs to meet the needs of the disabled and to begin to address these critical life issues.

The BOEC programs have served persons with cancer, hemophilia and epilepsy, individuals with impaired sight and hearing, and those with physical and developmental disabilities.

Since 1970, the National Sports Center for the Disabled at Winter Park, Colo., USA has provided recreational opportunities for disabled individuals. The program began with a group of amputee skiers from The Children's Hospital in Denver, and has expanded beyond the realm of recreational and competitive skiing. It also challenges the disabled year-round to achieve in the areas of rafting, climbing, and other endeavors. Through the National Sports Center for the Disabled at Winter Park, significant milestones have been made in the development of specialized equipment and teaching techniques for handicapped skiing [1].

Winter Park's philosophy is to offer challenges that will create personal growth, enhance family involvement, and allow participants to experience the outdoors on an equal basis with the able bodied. Through this, there is increased self-confidence, improved self-awareness, and development of skills that will last a lifetime.

Philosophy

Hospitals, especially those in metropolitan areas, often serve children from a wide geographic region with a variety of cultural backgrounds. These children return to their home towns where the community may not understand the full implication of their disability or illness. And, despite the 'hospital family's' effort to provide a warm and nurturing experience, the children may still return home feeling different than their peers, remembering a painful experience, fearing the future, and resenting the time taken away from being with family and friends.

At the core of the development of programs for children with special needs is the philosophy that a successful and challenging 'out of hospital' experience in sporting and recreation activities has a significant positive impact on the ability of these children to go on with their lives. Special programs for children with chronic illness and disabilities promote challenges and achievement without concern for the acceptance of others. The child is accepted into these programs for who he or she is, regardless of disability or illness. Self-image is enhanced through a sense of identity within this special group and the children take pride in their physical abilities, despite perceived limitations.

In summary, controlled and guided 'out of hospital' group activities for the handicapped facilitate acquisition of new skills, fulfillment of physical challenges, sharing of problems and special concerns, enhanced physical fitness, increased self-esteem, and development of strategies to deal with everyday problems.

Program Planning

Resources

Geographic location and existing community resources are key factors to consider in developing specialized therapeutic programs. The Children's Hospital in Denver, by virtue of its proximity to the Rocky Mountains, has access to recreational resources unique to mountain terrain. Additionally, community-based programs for special needs populations have flourished over the past two decades. Utilization of existing resources is beneficial since they provide programs with already established teaching techniques, adaptive equipment, and training programs.

Population

Most pediatric health care facilities have specialized inpatient and outpatient departments serving children with a variety of chronic diseases and handicapping conditions. Sports and recreational programs for these populations may be developed by individual departments, or the institution may choose to coordinate all special needs programs. Once particular needs are identified, program planners may develop special programs using the interests and expertise of staff members as well as resources available in the community. Programs may choose to limit involvement to their hospital's population or expand beyond institutional walls and invite participation of special needs children from other facilities.

Staff Needs/Requirements

All 'special needs' sports and recreation programs must have dedicated staff, committed to providing 'a little bit' extra to make these special programs possible. In many situations, this commitment is over and beyond the normal work hours. However, for the programs to function, volunteers are vital. Individual programs must determine volunteer requirements (i.e. activity skill level, training needs) and these requirements must be established in advance of program involvement. In larger programs, these guidelines need to be in written format.

Financing

Operation of all special needs programs is costly. Either the program owns and operates a recreational facility or it must contract for services with outside specialty resources. Special liability insurance may be purchased to supplement the institutional umbrella policy. Transportation costs, special dietary requirements, medical supplies and special equipment all contribute to the program costs. Medical staff members in some programs are paid; in other programs, professional staff fees are waived, but food and lodging must be provided. Financial assistance for participants with established need must be considered. Program souvenirs for the children, if not donated by a sponsor, must be included when estimating the program costs.

Grants, donations and fundraising events can provide much of the necessary financial support. Many programs charge nominal fees for participation. Although these fees may not cover program costs completely, they do help defray expenses and they have a significant impact on the interest and feeling of investment by the participants and their families.

Liability Issues

Involvement in recreation and sports activities is not without risk. With the handicapped, this risk may be higher than in the normal population. Children, whether able-bodied or disabled, lack sophisticated judgment skills and therefore require guidance in program participation. The handicapped child, competing with his able-bodied peers, may fail to recognize his limitations, thus making guidance/supervision essential.

An important element of program planning is obtaining legal advice regarding liability. Adequate insurance coverage is essential. Participation in a sanctioned hospital volunteer program may provide adequate liability coverage for volunteer staff, or group policies for special camps and activities may be available for purchase from specialty organizations. Special staff/volunteer training requirements may be required for liability protection. Volunteer liability releases should be considered. In all instances, parents/guardians of participating children must sign forms to release the program sponsor in matters of emergency care, transportation, photo and media matters, and risks of basic program participation.

Transportation

Most medical facilities have regulations established by their insurance carriers regarding chauffeuring of clients by staff and volunteers. These regulations should be examined carefully when program-sponsored transportation is considered. Although costly, contractual services with a public carrier for transportation should be taken into account.

Special Equipment Needs

Development of specialized equipment for the handicapped has flourished; some of this equipment is designed specifically for sporting activities. Specialized sporting equipment must be proven to be safe and must be maintained properly, with users adequately instructed in its use. Appropriate safety gear is essential.

In the ideal situation, each child would have the appropriate wheelchair, prosthesis, or orthotic device to use while engaging in an activity. However, many children require regular replacement of devices for growth and the additional expense of specialized sporting equipment is prohibitive for many families. Therefore, many children use their regular equipment in recreational activities; adaptation and precaution to preserve the life of the device(s) are imperative.

Participant Selection

Program goals and objectives determine the guidelines for participant selection. Sometimes a blend of disabilities or various levels of functioning work well together in one program, whereas participants with similar problems may enhance the quality of another program. Applicants must be assessed for their appropriateness for program participation by evaluating physical ability, level of social functioning and special needs. The success of any program depends on strong parental support for the children's participation. With proper selection of participants, program success and participant gains are maximized.

Thorough medical background information on each child is essential. These data must provide valuable information regarding the need for medical intervention and adaptive aids, precautions and/or contraindications to be considered, special staff/volunteer training needs, and behavior considerations. From this information, realistic expectations can be established for the child's participation.

Medical Needs

Crucial to program planning for outdoor experiences for special populations is the assessment, evaluation and provision for health and medical needs. An essential component is having thorough knowledge of the illness and disability and its impact on the individual.

Participant data collection and health histories assist in this process. In addition, there are many related factors that should not be overlooked. Figure 1 provides a guideline for key medical issues and needs which should be considered in program planning.

Specialty Programs and Camps

Professionals from The Children's Hospital in Denver participate in a variety of specialty programs and camps. Several such programs are discussed as examples of recreational and sporting programs for children with special needs.

A Wilderness Program for Adolescents with Cancer

Since 1981, groups of adolescents aged 12–24 years with cancer from The Children's Hospital have participated in winter and summer wilderness experiences at BOEC in Colorado. These adolescents were identified as a patient population who became isolated in the pediatric setting and were in need of a special program to address their needs.

Adolescents with cancer are faced with the devastating task of integrating the diagnosis of cancer and treatment with the complex developmental issues of adolescence. These teenagers must face the life-threatening nature of the disease as well as the chronicity of it. They must learn to contend with and develop coping skills to deal with treatment, side effects, complications and psychological sequelae. Some adolescents have described the treatment as worse than the disease. Struggles include a sense of being different and varying energy levels as well as changes in physical appearance due to hair loss, obesity, cachexia, or a physical disability like amputation. Socialization is of paramount importance during this time. Adolescents with cancer may face changes in peer relationships through loss, rejection, teasing, or time lost secondary to treatment. Treatment schedules are rigid and somewhat inflexible with respect to everyday life. In addition, adolescence is a time of emerging independence and these adolescents may never achieve

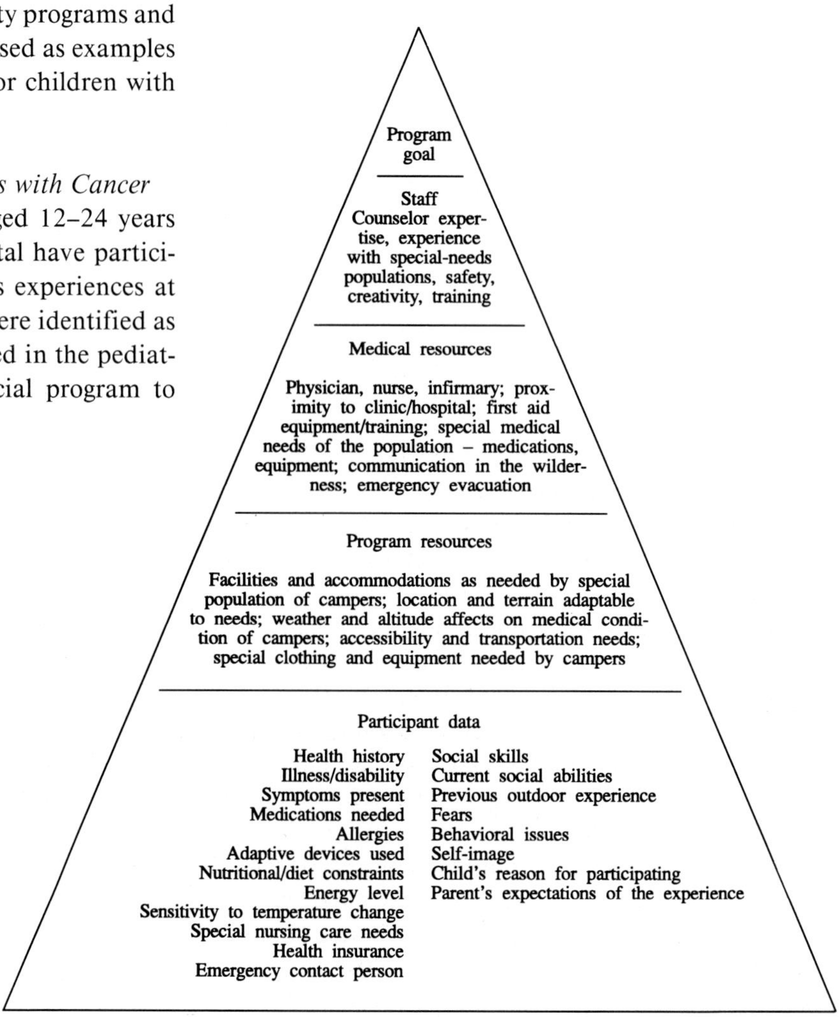

Fig. 1. Guideline for identification of health needs of specialty program participants.

autonomy or may have the process stunted due to the need to resume parental dependence. Parental concerns may result in overprotection and guilt. Social and financial stresses within the family may have an impact on the adolescent and may contribute to the overall experience.

While the program involves adolescents who are undergoing chemotherapy, often adolescents who have completed treatment participate as well. This mix provides a unique opportunity for individuals off treatment to serve as role models. It is valuable to 'see' those who 'have made it'. In addition, there exist underlying bonds of mutuality that encourage sharing, support and encouragement that otherwise might not happen.

Adolescent survivors often have unfinished work with their cancer, treatment, and its impact on their life. While completing treatment is a much desired milestone, it is only the first step in a rehabilitation that allows not only for cure but healing and realized potential growth.

With advances in cancer treatment, more adolescents diagnosed with cancer are living longer, and increasing numbers of children with cancer are surviving into adolescence. By the year 1990, one in every 1,000 adults will be a survivor of childhood cancer [2]. A major thrust in the care of cancer patients is to enhance their quality of life by minimizing the psychosocial consequences of treatment.

The program at BOEC is designed to offer activities such as rock climbing (fig. 2), river rafting, ropes course, nordic and alpine skiing, hiking, camping, back packing, wilderness survival, solo experience and sit skiing. Students progress through a series of challenges created to bring them to a level of stress, but also designed to guarantee success. Experientially, the students find they are capable of doing more physically and mentally than they thought possible. These successes are transferred to day-to-day life and result in empowerment. The setting is rustic without running water or electricity. Trust, sharing and community building serve as the framework for the program. To foster self-responsibility, students are given the opportunity to assume responsibility for medications unless supervision is required.

Therapeutic wilderness programming has proven to be a successful modality to challenge adolescents with cancer and provide tools and skills to help them move on with their lives. Programs such as this help these individuals move beyond the cancer experience and survival and assist them in returning to a full life with dignity and personal growth.

The Handicapped Sports Program for Physically Handicapped Children

In 1968, the Three Track Ski Club, a ski program for children from the Amputee Clinic at The Children's Hospital began as one of the first such programs for children in the United States. Today, the program has expanded and is known as The Children's Hospital Handicapped Sports Program. It now provides a variety of year-round outdoor sports and recreation activities for children with various physical disabilities.

The objective of The Children's Hospital Handicapped Sports Program is to introduce handicapped children to recreational activities in an environment out of the hospital which help rehabilitate them physically and emotionally. As E. Williams, the founder of the Three Track Ski Club stated in the video 'Two, Three Fasten Your Ski', the hospital 'can fit an amputee with a prosthesis and teach the child to walk or use the arm. But to fully rehabilitate them, they must be a part of the community'.

Fulfillment of physical challenges plays a vital role in the development of self-esteem and self-confidence. With improvement in both of these areas, handicapped children may have greater academic achievement, will discover life-long sporting activities to enjoy with family and friends, and will have far greater opportunities available to them in the future. Lastly, the children benefit from improved physical fitness and a pride in their abilities despite their handicap.

Many children with disabilities (especially those present at birth), are overly sheltered or protected by

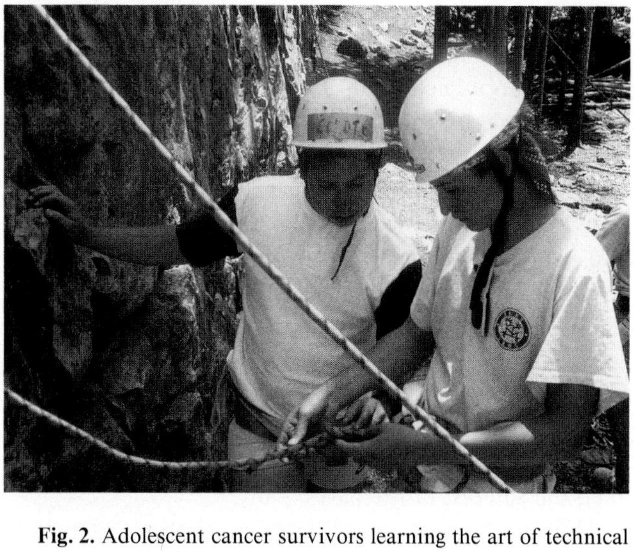

Fig. 2. Adolescent cancer survivors learning the art of technical rock climbing.

their families and often limited in their participation in physical activities in school and with their peers. The Children's Hospital Handicapped Sports Program provides a 'safe' environment which allows many families to 'let go' and permit their child's involvement in program activities.

This 'stepping stone' fosters additional involvement of the child in other community programs and promotes family involvement in activities that they may have thought impossible.

Although the Three Track Ski Club began with a small group of amputees, it was found that a blend of physical disabilities of children with similar functional levels (socially and physically) works well together. They help one another, their social realm expands, and they enjoy a special camaraderie not found in their mainstreamed world.

Disabilities of the children participants presently include cerebral palsy, spina bifida, amputation (congenital and acquired), poliomyelitis, arthrogryposis, head injury, and other orthopedic disabilities. Most of the children are referred to the program through the specialty clinics or medical staff at The Children's Hospital. Age ranges of participants are generally 8–18 years. Specific program requirements often determine the disability, functional level, and age range of the participants.

To participate in the program activities, children are encouraged to become more physically fit, acquire necessary skills of independence (i.e. bladder and bowel care), develop concern for pressure and frostbite of insensate skin, and successfully function socially within a peer group.

Over the years, The Handicapped Sports Program has offered a wide variety of activities: alpine and nordic skiing, sit skiing, tennis, river rafting, camping, golfing, bowling, horseback riding, and archery. The program activities are determined by the needs of the children as well as community resources available to the program.

In all the Handicapped Sports Program activities, the individual child's functional level (cognitively, socially and physically) is assessed and a positive experience is structured for the participant. Realistic expectations are established and equipment adaptations and/or special teaching techniques are determined. Although the initial goal is for the child to acquire some skill through participation, the activity must be directed toward having fun as well as providing a challenging element in order to keep the interest of the participant.

Horseback riding, one of the Handicapped Sports Program activities, allows the child to have a greater range of mobility throughout his/her environment as well as gaining a feeling of power brought about by controlling a large animal. Improvement in trunk stability and balance (fig. 3a, b), reduced tone in the child with spasticity, greater attention span, and improved communication skills are but a few of the gains noted in the horseback riding experience. During this activity, the skills of horsemanship are reinforced while specific activities are directed to enhance the child's physical abilities. The Children's Hospital Handicapped Program uses the resources of therapeutic riding programs in the community modeled after The Cheff Center in Michigan.

Skiing is the largest endeavor of the Handicapped Sports Program at The Children's Hospital. Downhill skiing produces movement through the assistance of gravity. This movement enables handicapped children to experience fluidity and grace of movement that does not exist in their everyday world. To best use this movement, equipment and teaching techniques are greatly modified. There are many variables to consider in adapting to meet the needs of the physically handicapped skier: discrepancy in extremity size, use of an orthotic or prosthetic device, abnormal posturing and tone with movement, diminished sensation and lack of muscle function/strength.

The Children's Hospital Handicapped Ski Program has participated at the Winter Park National Sports Center for the Disabled since 1970. Other special needs programs in community are used by the Handicapped Sports Program to provide additional recreational opportunities for program participants. In making the selection of the resource/facility to utilize, strong consideration is given as to whether it can provide a safe environment for the children and has established credibility in the given activity.

Volunteer assistance is a significant part of the operation of The Handicapped Sports Program. Since a variety of handicaps are included in the program activities, it is essential that the volunteers and instructors are knowledgeable about these disabilities. In addition, each child has his/her own special needs, and these needs must be made apparent to the responsible individuals. Instructor volunteers working with The Children's Hospital Handicapped Ski Program must be qualified through The National Sports Center for the Disabled at Winter Park. This is required to ensure the safety of the participant and to guarantee that each volunteer has the necessary skills and ability for this role. Extensive training at the onset of their involvement and periodic refresher clinic attendance are required. The variety of instructional methods (fig. 4)

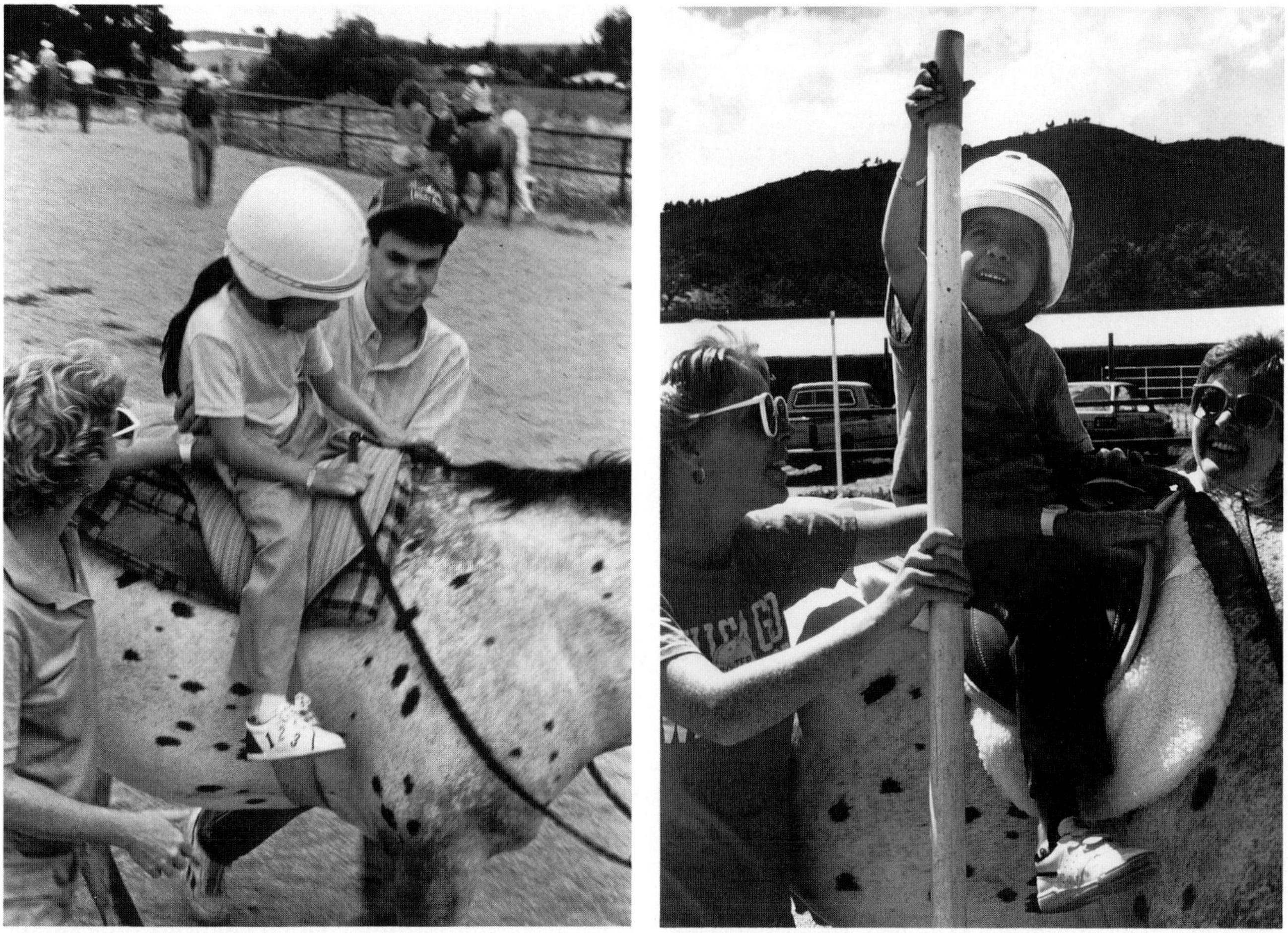

a b

Fig. 3. Therapeutic horseback riding. **a** Participant with spastic quadriplegia/cerebral palsy has slumped posture. **b** Improved posture attained with therapeutic activity.

used in the ski program necessitates these volunteer instructors being well versed in multiple areas.

Unique to The Handicapped Sports Program is the volunteer assistance of many adults with physical impairments as well as adults from the medical community. Many of the handicapped adults were participants in the program when they were younger and are eager to 'give something back to the program'. They are inspirational role models for the participants. Additionally, there is a great sense of 'normalizing' between medical staff volunteers and participants that cannot be achieved within the confines of the hospital environment.

Epilepsy Camp

Children 10–16 years old with epilepsy referred from the Neurology Department at The Children's Hospital have been participating in a wilderness experience at the BOEC since 1983.

This outdoor experience developed from recognition of the special needs of children with epilepsy. Children with seizure disorders may experience rejection and limitations through parental and societal fear. There is a fear of seizures – they are an 'invisible handicap' which occur unpredictably. These children are often excluded from regular camp programs because of their seizures. Eventually they do not participate because they have received the message they are not capable. They learn to be cautious as opposed to taking risk. This is a message which does not enhance growth and self-image.

The program at the BOEC deals with issues of safety, trust, and perceived risk. The activities assist participants to feel competent and in charge of their life. There is an opportunity to move from the feeling of helplessness and needing someone to take care of them to coping. This sense of coping is important especially when the 'unpredictable' event of a seizure occurs. For many

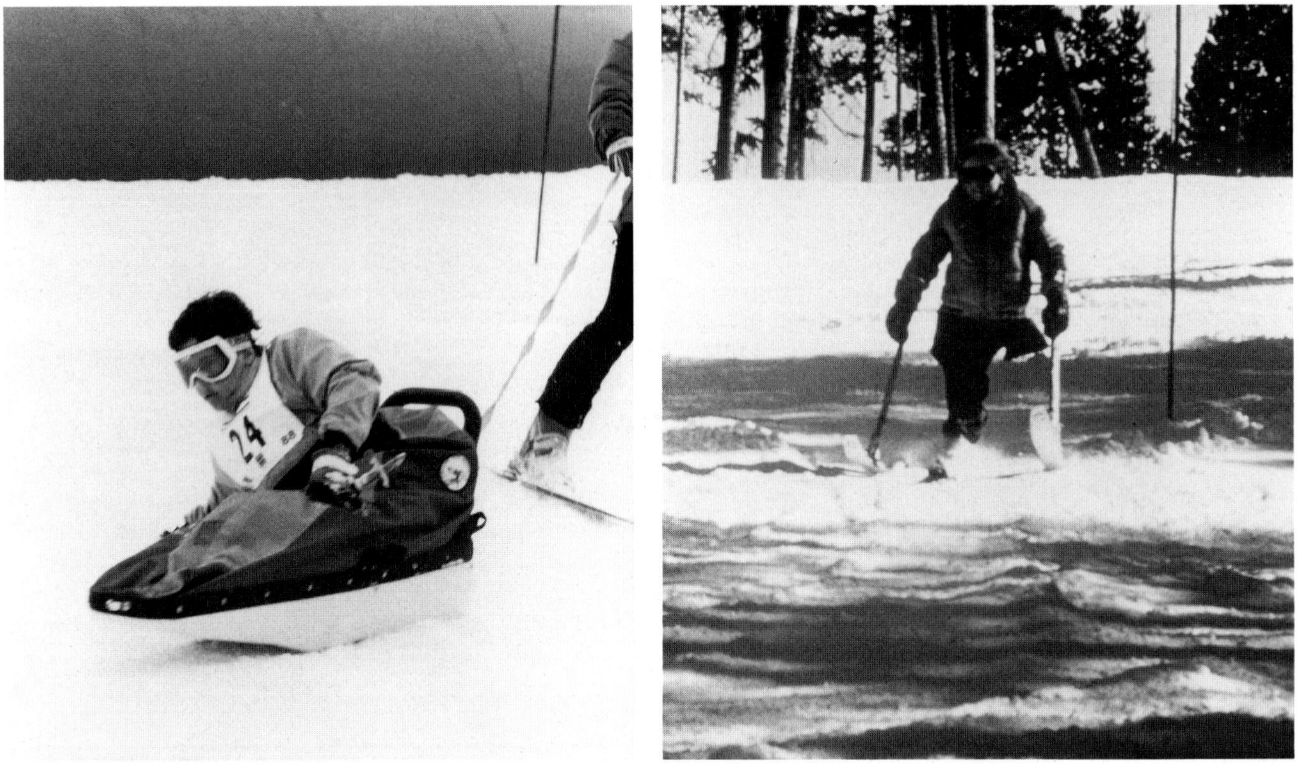

a b

Fig. 4. Therapeutic skiing. **a** Sit-skiing participant. **b** Amputee skier.

participants, this is the first time they see an actual seizure. A seizure is a 'normalizing event', decreasing fear of the unknown. In addition, it helps to bridge the gap of fears between the child who has a seizure problem and another person who is viewing the seizure for the first time. They learn how to help one another understand seizures. This sharing includes hearing from the person who had the seizure, what was done for them, what could have been done better, and how people responded. This experience enables the participants to be more comfortable with their seizures, teaches them how to handle them, and what to do to decrease fears.

The social worker for the program serves as a chaperone and also assumes the responsibility for giving medications and keeping a medical log. This individual actively participates in the program by assisting participants with their feelings regarding their seizure disorder.

Burn Camp

School age children with thermal injuries are a special population who benefit from a camp experience. These children often suffer severe injuries and struggle with self-esteem and identity issues. Frequently they are the only persons with burn scars in their school and community. There exists a lack of mental health professionals comfortable with and competent in treating the disfigured child.

In 1983, staff from the Burn Center at The Children's Hospital established a national camp to address the comprehensive, ongoing rehabilitation need of pediatric burn patients. The nature of the camp environment fosters staff-patient relationships and interactions away from the sterile image of the hospital where painful wound care procedures occur. The camp also allows for a therapeutic environment to emerge which sets the stage for 'on the spot' counselling around life issues for the child. In addition, staff develop a greater awareness of what it is like to live with burn scars and thus further establish their commitment to long-term rehabilitation of the pediatric burn patient.

The resources at Camp Cheley in Estes Park (Colo., USA) provide traditional programming (fig. 5) as well as special activities such as square dancing, puppetry, photography, and make-up/color lessons to enhance appearance.

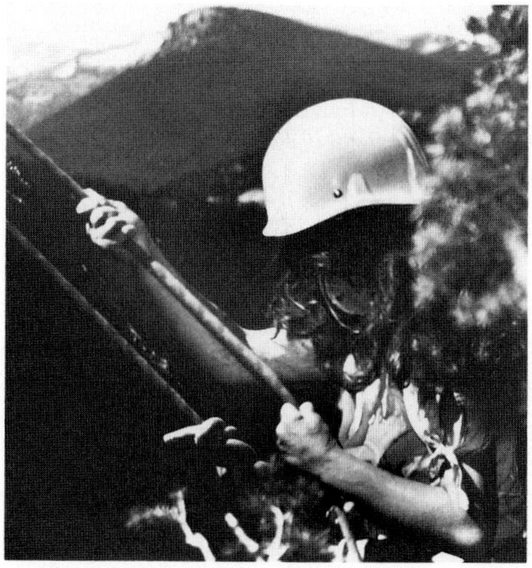

Fig. 5. Burn camp participant involved in technical rope climbing despite severe, deforming hand injuries.

Cheley camp and volunteer staff are integrated with professional staff from burn centers around the country. Nurses, occupational and physical therapists and psychotherapeutic staff (social work and child psychiatry) are available to meet the special needs of the campers. Burn physicians visit during the week to address any medical needs as well as to engage in camp activities.

The burn population often includes patients with premorbid social, emotional and academic dysfunction. The staff at The Children's Hospital Burn Camp has developed a thorough intake/screening process to identify appropriate candidates for the camp program and allow optimal preparation for individual camper needs. Parents and teachers as well as the various therapists, physicians and nurses from referring burn centers provide valuable information for precamp screening and selection of the camp participants. In addition, the Achenbach Child Behavior Checklist [3] is administered to parents and teachers to identify any specific problem areas not communicated through the family data and medical history forms. The expenditure of administrative time precamp allows the staff to offer optimum care as well as a safe, therapeutic camping experience. The philosophy of the Burn Camp staff is summarized: 'Children's Hospital has a strong conviction that to save children's lives is not enough. We are committed to help them face tomorrow and the rest of their lives.' (Marion Doctor, MSW, The Children's Hospital, the Burn Center, Denver, Colo.).

Sky-High Hope Camp for Children with Cancer

Sky-High Hope Camp was established in 1981 for children with cancer. Modeled after camps for children with cancer that originated in Florida, Illinois, and Michigan, this camp was based on the observation that children with cancer were unable to attend regular camp programs because of the impact of the disease and their physical and emotional needs. A camping opportunity was identified at The Children's Hospital as a means of support and socialization as well as reducing the isolation and loneliness that often were observed in children with cancer.

The camp medical program includes an infirmary staffed with a physician, a nurse, and a laboratory technician. The medical staff is prepared to handle any medical situation from routine upset stomachs, headaches, and insect bites to oncologic emergencies. The focus of the camp is on making the environment safe and normal as opposed to bringing the hospital to camp. The staff is equipped to give some chemotherapy orally, intramuscularly, or intravenously as long as it involves only an overnight stay in the infirmary at the most and does not interfere with the camping experience for the child.

Staff includes volunteers from all walks of life. Senior citizens and teachers are a good resource for volunteers in addition to medical staff volunteers. Parents are not directly involved in the camp to allow the children to separate and gain exposure to many different kinds of people. Therefore, both parents and children have an opportunity for separation, growth, and rejuvenation.

Diabetes Camp

Camps for children with diabetes serve a dual purpose: (1) to provide informal education in management skills, and (2) to provide a regular fun-filled camping experience for children who may be unable to attend regular camping programs.

Prior to camp, it is most important to obtain a good health history on each child. This information must include current insulin requirements, nutritional habits and recent blood glucose control.

An important component of the program is the education of nonmedical staff regarding hypoglycemia and the need for scheduled meals and snacks. A knowledgeable dietician is essential for meal planning and preparation of food. Medical staff should be adequate in number and experience to assist campers in adjusting insulin dosage and food intake to meet the rigors of increased activity.

For the child with diabetes, this camping experience may be the only contact with other children who have the same disorder. Fear and loneliness are defused through sharing common experiences. Some children with diabetes may develop a manipulative life style using their illness for control and/or attention. These cycles may change at camp where the child learns more effective coping patterns.

Diabetes camp often provides a much needed break for children and parents from each other. Children who have been overprotected can learn to do many things provided they want to plan for food and insulin adjustments. Parents enjoy a brief respite from the daily routine of timed meals, snacks, blood testing and injections.

Camp is a learning process for staff, too. Health personnel learn how and why children are noncompliant. They also develop a more realistic sense of what it is like to live with diabetes and understand how to manage children with diabetes more effectively.

Conclusion

Providing medical care for children and adolescents with chronic illness and disabilities often begins at the hospital. However, rehabilitation is an integral part of the care of the child which fosters return to wholeness and optimal function. Wholeness requires acceptance and integration of the illness or disability by the child, family, school, and community.

Recreational, sports and therapeutic camping experiences are tools that can enhance the rehabilitation and healing of a child. These programs may be pioneered through the efforts of committed hospital staff who believe in the rich and therapeutic nature of these experiences for a child with chronic illness or a disability.

In addition to the positive impact on the child, these programs offer hospital staff the opportunity to share the child's vulnerability, as well as give time and support to these children. There is a sense of mutuality through which staff and children get to know one another outside the hospital, and learn about each other. Staff has the first-hand opportunity to see and experience the impact of the illness or disability on the child's life. This 'hands on' experience generates enhanced care and understanding.

These programs invite the opportunity to reach toward a common goal: caring for individuals who touch our lives in a most profound way.

Appendix

A partial list of resources used by The Children's Hospital Camp and Recreational Programs for handicapped and chronically ill children (listed below in *alphabetical order*).

American Diabetes Association: 1660 Duke Street, Alexandria, VA 22314
Advisory committee for diabetes camping.

Breckenridge Outdoor Education Center (BOEC): PO Box 697, Breckenridge, CO 80404. (303) 453-6424

Cheff Center for the Handicapped: Augusta, Mich. (Well-known North American training center for horseback riding for the handicapped)

Aspects and Answers: A Manual for Therapeutic Horseback Riding Programs (1986): Joswick, Kittredge, McCowan, McPharland, Woods. Direct inquiries to: Executive Director, Cheff Center, Augusta, MI 49012

The Children's Hospital Burn Camp: The Children's Hospital, Burn Center, 1056 E. 19th Ave., Denver, CO 80218. (303) 861-8888

High Road to Recovery: a 13-min video featuring The Children's Hospital Burn Camp. US$60.00. Direct inquiries to The Children's Hospital Burn Center.

Children's Oncology Camps of America (COCA): Children's Memorial Hospital, 2300 Children's Plaza, Chicago, IL 60614. (312) 880-4564

Crystal Productions, Inc.: Box 2159, Glenview, IL 60025. (312) 657-8144 (outside of Illinois 1-800-255-8629)
Distributor of Rehabilitation Films

The Children's Hospital, Denver, Colo.: Handicapped Sports Program Films
- No Simple Road: a 16-min film/video featuring children with a variety of physical disabilities enjoying many year around recreational/sporting activites.
- The Mountain Does It For Me: a 12-min film/video featuring children with cerebral palsy learning to ski in The Children's Hospital downhill ski program.
- Two, Three Fasten Your Ski: a 17-min film/video showing amputee children participating in The Children's Hospital Three Track Ski Club.

The Children's Hospital, Denver, Colo.: Oncology Department Films
- Childhood Cancer: Patients Speak Out: a 16-min film/video featuring children with cancer who share their feelings and are shown participating in normal activities.
- Children Cancer: Siblings Speak Out: a 22-min film/video used as a clinical tool to assist families of children with cancer and other chronic illnesses.

NHSRA / National Handicapped Sports and Recreation Association / National Handicapped Sports (1989): 1145 19th St. NW Suite 717, Washington, DC 20036. (301) 652-7505
National sports and recreational organization supporting the handicapped with many regional chapters throughout the United States.

Never Say Never: 1309 E. Northern No. 308, Phoenix, AZ 85020: A video demonstrating golf for the physically challenged.

Sports and Recreation for the Disabled: A Resource Handbook, Paciorek MJ, Jones JA: Specialized Sports Unlimited. Indianapolis, Benchmark Press, 1989.

Sports 'N Spokes: 5201 N. 19th Ave. Suite 111. Phoenix, AZ 85015 (602) 249-9426
A bimonthly magazine representing wheelchair competitive sports and recreation primarily for those with spinal cord injury, spina bifida, amputation, and some congenital defects.

Sunshine Kids Foundation: c/o Rhoda Tomasco, 3228 Reba Drive, Houston, TX 77019
Sponsor of special programs for children with cancer

Textbook of Sports for the Disabled: Guttman Sir L. Aylesbury, HM & M Publishers, 1976.

Winter Park Resort: National Sports Center for the Disabled, PO Box 36, Winter Park, CO 80482. (303) 726-5514

Winter Park Handicap Program: Hal O'Leary PSIA, Director.

Winter Park Competition Center for Disabled Athletes: Paul DiBello, Director.

Bold Tracks/Skiing for the Disabled: O'Leary H. Evergreen, Cordillera Press, 1987.

References

1 O'Leary H: Bold Tracks/Skiing for the Disabled. Evergreen, Cordillera Press, 1987.
2 Meadows AT: Delayed consequences of therapy for childhood cancer. Cancer J Clin 1985;35:271–286.
3 Achenbach TM: Child Behavior Checklist. Bethesda, National Institute of Mental Health, 1979.

Received: October 15, 1989

Carol J. Page, RPT
Handicapped Sports Program
Department of Physical Therapy
The Children's Hospital
Denver, CO 80218 (USA)

Pediatrician 1990;17:308–313

Transition of the Disabled Adolescent to Adulthood

Charlotte E. Thompson

Center for Handicapped Children and Teenagers, San Francisco, Calif.;
Department of Pediatrics, University of California Medical School, San Diego, Calif., USA

Key Words. Adolescent · Disabled adolescent · Independence, steps to · Medical management · Social skills · Counseling

Abstract. Disabled teenagers have problems making the transition from adolescence to adulthood. Helping parents, particularly mothers, 'let go' is an important part of the medical management, as is coordinating the complex medical, social, and educational aspects. Issues of bowel and bladder care, sexuality, dating, dressing, and driving must be considered. Role modeling by successful disabled adults and counseling assist in successful transition.

Making the transition from adolescence to adulthood is difficult enough without the added problem of a disability. Complications multiply if the parents have problems allowing self-sufficiency or the nature of the disability hinders independence. A major responsibility for those who work with parents is to encourage them to gradually 'let go' of their children and to monitor that this process is occurring [1]. Knowing when it is appropriate to increase a young person's responsibilities and level of independence is difficult for parents (and sometimes for professionals), particularly if the youth's disability causes growing incapacity. The current prevalence of kidnapping, child abuse, and other crimes adds to the difficulty of allowing children much freedom. Disabled children and teenagers are particularly at risk if they are physically limited and can neither run from potential harm nor try to defend themselves. Teenagers with developmental delay may be unable to evaluate a situation or individual and thus be unaware of possible danger.

Parents should begin to teach children to become independent adults in their early years by delegating more and more responsibilities. Having daily chores appropriate for their abilities, learning to manage money, and having to make decisions are ways to develop independence. Involving children in planning what they can do is important, too. Disabled children are often catered to by all members of the family and not allowed or expected to shoulder their share of responsibilities. It is usually much easier for parents and others to do things for handicapped children or teenagers without giving them the opportunity to try. This is particularly true now that the majority of parents work outside the home. Time and energy have become precious commodities, and finding the time or patience to wait while a disabled child undertakes a task may just not be possible, unless some planning and rethinking are done.

Mothers of disabled children may become such an important force in their children's lives that they even speak for them. Thus, when examining children or teenagers, we must allow them to speak for themselves as much as possible. All health care personnel should be encouraged to do this; if necessary, parents should be asked to wait in the reception area. All individuals should be able to discuss their own medical problems and feelings with physicians. Without opportunities to do this, teenagers may withdraw into protective shells and allow parents and others to communicate for them. The less they try or the less they are given the opportunity, the more difficult communicating becomes. Communication with teenagers is difficult for many adults; both professionals and parents should use every means possible to keep the channels open. Dependence breeds anger in anyone, and in a disabled individual this can add to the anger that may be present because of the handicap. Counseling can be an important tool in helping a teenager make the necessary transition from adolescence to maturity. It may be difficult to find a counselor who truly understands an adolescent's pain, but disabled counselors can act as role models and smooth the transition to adulthood. Peer counseling and interacting with support groups can also help as can role modeling by successful disabled adults.

The high divorce and separation rates among parents of disabled children are well known. Parents should be encouraged to have lives of their own apart from their disabled teenagers. By having time for themselves, they will find it easier both to allow their teenager more independence and to put more energy into preserving their own relationship.

Adolescent Sexuality

Discussion of sexuality is very important with adolescents, but it must be handled with great tact and gentleness, particularly if the youth has spina bifida, paraplegia, or other central nervous system dysfunction. Sex and disability counselors are available in many areas through medical schools or rehabilitation facilities.

If the teenager has cerebral palsy with athetosis or muscular dystrophy with progressive weakness, other problems in handling sexuality can arise. The inability to touch and interact in a normal adult manner can be devastating, and other methods must be taught so that warmth and love can be given and received. No one can live without some touching and warmth. Because a disabled teenager so often feels isolated, the absence of normal sexual interaction can increase this feeling. Discussions of sexual feelings and fantasies should be held with trained professionals comfortable with these topics.

Developing Full Potential

Helping disabled teenagers develop their greatest potential is important to their becoming mature, capable adults. Special education when necessary should begin in the early years. Present federal legislation is making it easier to obtain; however, parents and professionals must work together as a team to ensure the best possible program for each individual child. The bureaucracy has increasingly regulated the education of disabled children and youth without adding sufficient personnel or money to fulfill the legislative requirements.

Measuring a child's ability by a battery of psychometric tests early on its important [1, 2]. This testing must be done by a skilled educational psychologist accustomed to testing disabled children. Testing on just one occasion may not be adequate; it may need to be repeated every 2–3 years. A child's individual educational plan (IEP) should be carefully worked out by a team to reflect the test results and provide the best education possible. If children and teenagers can be involved in developing some of their own goals in and out of school, they usually feel more a part of the process and thus put more energy into achieving these goals.

The decision whether or not to mainstream a teenager can be a difficult one. If there is a specific disability, such as blindness or deafness, specialized training is needed and may have to be provided in a residential setting, although the necessary funding for this may be hard to secure.

As nondisabled children and teenagers in regular school programs can be very cruel, educating both the school personnel and students prior to admitting a disabled youth is important. Painful stories of teasing, isolation, and actual physical harm have been told by disabled students who were the only handicapped individual in a regular classroom. Getting these students involved in classroom activities to the maximum of their ability and stressing their areas of competence are vital. Not knowing how best to handle a disability, classmates and teachers often keep the disabled child or adolescent at a distance in the back of the room, with resultant increased loneliness and isolation.

Physicians and other health care professionals should be involved in explaining particular disabilities to both

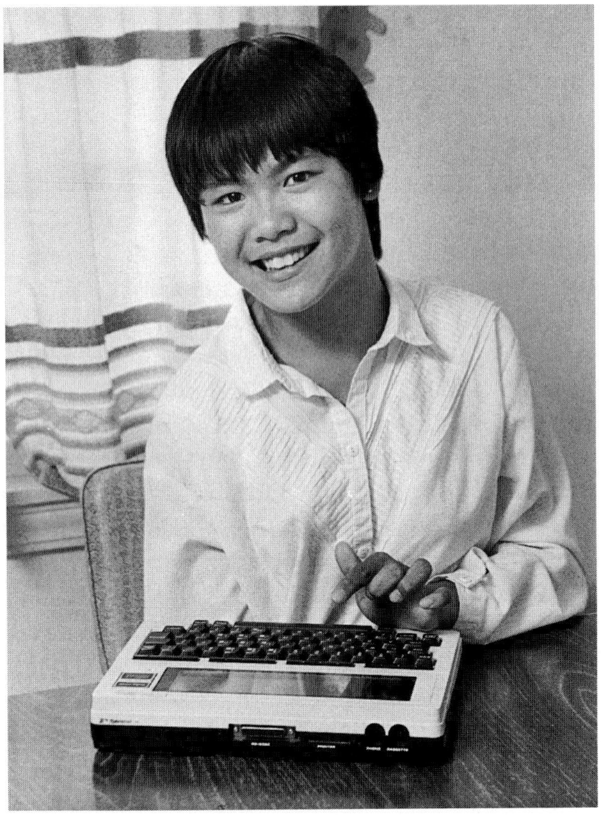

Fig. 1. Cerebral palsy teenager using small desktop computer for communication purposes.

school personnel and pupils. Unfortunately, little of this seems to occur, and there is often little communication between school personnel and the medical team. Many IEP teams neither notify the involved medical personnel nor particularly like to have them present when IEPs are created. Yet as children and teenagers with more complex medical problems attend regular schools, physicians, in particular, should be involved in helping to plan their curricula. Youth with complex medical problems often are cared for by teachers and aides who have no in-service training about the medical condition. Periodic conversations with school personnel should be part of the medical management of the disabled teenager.

When learning disabilities are present, one-to-one help frequently is needed in a classroom. Identifying the learning disabilities early on is extremely important so that the special assistance can be obtained. Spina bifida and Duchenne dystrophy patients have an especially high incidence of learning disabilities which should be looked for in the early school years [3, 4]. The 'chatterbox' speech often seen in spina bifida children and teenagers may make them appear much brighter than they are [3]. Thus, psychometric tests should be done in the early school years to determine their actual abilities so that plans for any needed special help can be made.

If children have been in a school for the orthopedically handicapped, the emphasis may have been on physical and occupational therapy rather than on academic learning. Many of these children are then mainstreamed in their adolescent years and simply do not have the educational tools to keep up with their nondisabled peers. This results in a poor self-image and increased isolation.

Computers are proving to be of tremendous value to many disabled children and youths (fig. 1). Having their own computer at school can mean the difference between achieving or falling behind. It may also facilitate the transition to adulthood and work because computer skills are so much in demand. Many adaptive devices are available for individuals with limited motor ability, and every effort should be made to see that these are available to patients [5].

Community skills should be taught in all programs for developmentally delayed and physically handicapped adolescents. These can be written into the young peoples' IEPs. Trips to stores or shopping malls, use of community transportation, and learning how to order in restaurants are all important in making a smooth transition from adolescence to adulthood. What can be achieved is, of course, dependent on each individual's potential.

With a progressive neuromuscular disorder and resultant increased weakness or disability, marked changes may occur that make adulthood an even more difficult and dependent time. Depression is a frequent problem and can interfere with function and achievement. Hope must never be taken away; medical research and technology are developing tools that will both prolong and improve the quality of life.

Social Life

Friends are important to all of us, but particularly to disabled teenagers. Many parents restrict their disabled children and teenagers to friendships with nondisabled youth. This limits their choices, and having few friends may cause depression and withdrawal. Young persons in wheelchairs may be limited in their opportunities to interact, so any possible means for socialization should be encouraged. Clubs, camps, church groups, and special recreation programs all offer opportunities for finding friends. Sometimes, too, an electric wheelchair rather than a manual one can make a real difference in independence, allowing users to visit friends and be more in control of their lives.

Teenage peer groups are important, too. Often an interested school counselor or youth leader can be asked to help form a group and keep it going. Long-term friendships can be established, and the experience can make a lifelong impact.

Dating, driving, and dressing are three important Ds of adolescence. If a teenager has the intellectual capacity to drive and needs adaptive devices put on a car to make this possible, all effort should be made to accomplish this. The Department of Rehabilitation may help with vans and adaptive devices for cars if the car is used to find and keep employment. However, families interested in obtaining this type of financial aid should begin 2–3 years before the anticipated date of need because the paperwork is voluminous, and the energy required to obtain assistance is usually considerable.

Opportunities for dating should be encouraged when appropriate. Grooming and social skills should be taught, and any needed special clothing should be obtained. Many teenagers with physical disabilities find that members of the opposite sex often are put off by crutches and wheelchairs. One young man with flail lower legs from polio said that because he used crutches, the girls thought he was 'funny in the head' and stayed away from him. Constant rejection may necessitate counseling; health professionals should observe disabled adolescents closely for depression.

Employment

Special work programs may be not only a way to develop job skills, but also a way to make friends and increase social skills. Job training and career counseling are extremely important for disabled teenagers [6]. Some states have excellent college programs providing transportation, aides, and job training. The Department of Rehabilitation, Goodwill Industries, and Salvation Army all are sources for adult employment. However, finding a job through the Department of Rehabilitation may be a long, arduous task, and a great deal of stamina is required to use these facilities.

Private, nonprofit agencies, such as Careers Abound in San Francisco, are often preferable alternatives. Careers Abound, for example, helps prepare physically disabled teenagers for the world of work. They use grant funds and private donations to provide work experience opportunities, career counseling, and skills training. This makes the transition into the work force much easier and gives physically disabled youth needed skills and job confidence.

Aides and Role Models

Because government monies can be obtained for aides when a youth has severe disabilities, discussion of what type of aide they need must be raised with families. Often a parent, particularly the mother, will be paid as the aide, increasing the symbiotic relationship between mother and teenager. Teenage boys, in particular, need male attendants and should not always have their mothers with them. These male attendants often act as friends, too, thus widening the young person's circle. Having a parent always in attendance does a teenager a real disservice and does not allow the parent to have a life of his or her own.

Disabled adults can play an important part in the lives of these teenagers. Having a successful disabled adult as a role model gives a teenager hope for the future [6, 7]. Practical information about surmounting hurdles can also be shared, making a very positive experience for both the disabled youth and the adult. Adult male role modeling is vital for the children of single-parent mothers, and using the Big Brother organization and male relatives and friends is important for both boys and girls.

Health Care

A major medical problem for disabled teenagers today is that once they have outgrown pediatric care, few adult physicians are interested or equipped to provide needed care. Thus, many disabled young adults are still being cared for by their pediatricians. As more disabled adults are insisting on good medical care, specialty physicians or clinics may develop. However, currently few family physicians or internists are interested in coordinating the complex medical problems of disabled individuals. Such coordination can become a real financial burden for physicians if they take the necessary amount of time for it. Reimbursement by most state programs is extremely poor, and insurance companies do not pay for the time-consuming efforts of conferences and telephone coordination.

Medical care for disabled children and youth is also becoming more fragmented in many areas. Patients often are seen in large specialty clinics with little communication between the pediatrician or family physician and the clinic doctors. Some parents are asked to take their children and teenagers to several different specialists who do not communicate. Much overlap of services can occur, or routine procedures such as blood counts, urinalysis, tuberculin skin tests, and immunizations may be overlooked.

Spina bifida and spinal cord injury patients need a urological review at least every 2 years to be sure no kidney damage is occurring. Urine cultures should be done when there is increased urinary frequency, leaking, or odor. The question of maintenance antibiotics needs to be discussed with the urologist, and fluid intake should be carefully monitored because teenagers are generally poor about this, particularly if it necessitates more frequent catheterization.

Every attempt should be made to get children and teenagers out of diapers, using collection devices and leg bags for boys and ureostomies or a program of self-catheterization for girls [8]. (Catheterization in boys often is poorly accepted.) Self-catheterization can begin as early as age 5 with a bright, willing little girl. The earlier it is initiated, the easier it will be to establish and maintain an ongoing program. If catheterization has not been started at an early age or is not successful later on, a ureostomy may be the best answer. Having an older teenager show his or her collecting bag and ostomy to a younger one is often helpful to both.

A bowel program [9] should begin when the child is 2 or 3 years of age to be sure it is working successfully by the school years. There is nothing more difficult for a child and classmates to endure than obvious fecal smell. Children can be severely ostracized by their peers and others when there is a constant odor.

Teenagers who have never been put on a good program of bowel management may find it difficult to establish one. In addition, there may be a strong emotional component associated with diapers in older children and teenagers that even counseling cannot undo. A teenager's self-image can be severely impacted if he or she still wears diapers. Physicians who allow this to occur are doing a real disservice to their patients and should make every effort to establish a good bowel and bladder program [9]. Colostomies can be created surgically if a high-fiber diet, adequate fluid and protein, and suppositories properly used do not control the bowels.

Because some teenagers with chronic illness may be hospitalized frequently, the hospital may become a 'safe place', and this dependency may be hard to undo. One teenager with spina bifida who had little parenting either consciously or unconsciously became impacted every few months to make hospitalization necessary. The hospital was truly the only place she could be completely dependent, and the doctors and nurses essentially became her 'family'.

The onset of menstruation can be a real burden to some teenage girls who physically cannot cope with their menstrual flow. Their parents may raise the question of sterilization, and the involved physicians need to have consultation readily available by gynecologists and psychiatrists trained to discuss the moral and ethical issues involved. The possibility of early unwanted pregnancies is a real fear for many parents of severely disabled teenage girls, and discussion of prevention must be routine for physicians working with these patients. Parents become particularly concerned when these teenagers are institutionalized or placed in foster homes.

Clothing can be adapted to handle bowel, bladder, and menstrual problems, and parents can obtain catalogues from specialized clothing firms. Because appropriate dress is particularly important to teenage girls, parents should make every effort to find clothing that can be adapted to their needs. For example, velcro fasteners are useful for cerebral palsy patients and others with limited hand function [10].

Conclusion

Adolescence can be a time of many peaks and valleys. Without the ongoing help and guidance of trained, caring professionals, life can become an emotional roller coaster ride for both disabled young people and their parents. Anger, depression and even estrangement may occur. Professionals working together as a team with the parents and the adolescents can make the difference in keeping things under control so that creativity, self-sufficiency, feelings of competency and finally maturity can be fostered. The results can be extremely gratifying to all.

References

1 Thompson, C.E.: Raising a handicapped child (Ballantine, New York 1987).
2 Leonard, C.O.: Counseling parents of a child with meningocoele. Pediat. Rev. *4:* 317–321 (1983).
3 Raimondi, A.J.; Soare, P.: Intellectual development in shunted hydrocephalic children. AJDC *127:* 664 –671 (1974).

4 Marsh, G.G.; Munsat, T.: Evidence for early impairment of verbal intelligence in Duchenne muscular dystrophy. Archs Dis. Childh. *49:* 118–122 (1974).
5 Bigge, J.: Teaching individuals with physical and multiple disabilities (Merrill, Columbus 1982).
6 Blum, R.W.: The adolescent with spina bifida. Clin. Pediat. *22:* 331–335 (1983).
7 Hayden, P.W.; Davenport, S.L.H.; Campbell, M.M.: Adolescents with myelodysplasia: impact of physical disability on emotional maturation. Pediatrics *64:* 53–58 (1979).
8 Lyon, R.P.; Scott, M.P.: Intermittent catheterization rather than urinary diversion in children with meningocoele. J. Urol. *113:* 409–417 (1975).
9 Downey, J.A.; Low, N.L.: The child with disabling illness (Saunders, Philadelphia 1974).
10 Goldsworthy, M.: Clothes for disabled people (Batsford, London 1981).

Received: May 22, 1989

Charlotte E. Thompson, MD
Suite 307
2000 Van Ness Avenue
San Francisco, CA 94109 (USA)

Author Index

Subject Index

Announcement

4th International Symposium on Pediatric Dermatology

Mazara del Vallo (Trapani), Italy – September 25–28, 1991

Organized by the Gaspare Morello International Center for Study and Research and the Foundation for Research in Dermatology

Honorary President: Ferdinando Serri, MD
President: Decio Cerimele, MD
Topics:

- The role of the mass media in pediatric dermatology
- AIDS in children
- Mycoses in pediatric patients
- Nevi and melanomas in children
- Alopecia in children
- Ichthyoses and prenatal diagnosis
- Psychosomatic factors in atopic dermatitis
- Bullous diseases in children
- Acne
- Rare dermatological conditions in children

Official languages: English, Italian, French (simultaneous translation will be provided)

For further information please contact:

Giuseppe Fabrizi, MD
Scientific Program Director
Department of Dermatology
Catholic University
Largo Gemelli, 8
I-00168 Rome (Italy)
Telephone 06-33054227/33054211

Vol. 17, 1990

Pediatrician

International Journal of Child and Adolescent Health

Founded 1858 as 'Jahrbuch für Kinderheilkunde und physische Erziehung', continued as 'Annales Paediatrici' (1938–1966), 'Pediatric Research' (1967–1970) and 'Paediatrician' (1972–1982)

1890 1990 KARGER

KARGER

S. Karger · Medical and Scientific Publishers
Basel · München · Paris · London · New York · New Delhi · Bangkok · Singapore · Tokyo · Sydney

Drug Dosage

The authors and the publisher have exerted every effort to ensure that drug selection and dosage set forth in this text are in accord with current recommendations and practice at the time of publication. However, in view of ongoing research, changes in government regulations, and the constant flow of information relating to drug therapy and drug reactions, the reader is urged to check the package insert for each drug for any change in indications and dosage and for added warnings and precautions. This is particularly important when the recommended agent is a new and/or infrequently employed drug.

Printed in Switzerland by Thür AG Offsetdruck, Pratteln

Contents Vol. 17, 1990

No. 1

Sleep Disorders in Childhood and Adolescence

No. 2

Ethical Problems in Pediatrics

No. 3

Ophthalmic Disorders of Children

No. 4

Pediatric Rehabilitation